Keto Diet C

Beginners

A Comprehensive Guide to Jumpstart Your
Ketogenic Journey and Achieve Optimal
Health and Weight Loss

By Ryann Barbara

TABLE OF CONTENTS

Welcome to the "Keto Diet Cookbook For Beginners: A Comprehensive Guide to Jumpstart Your Ketogenic Journey and Achieve Optimal Health and Weight Loss." Whether you're new to the ketogenic diet or looking to refresh your knowledge, this ebook is here to guide you through the exciting and transformative process of adopting a keto lifestyle.

The ketogenic diet has gained tremendous popularity in recent years due to its ability to promote weight loss, improve mental clarity, increase energy levels, and enhance overall well-being. By shifting your body into a state of ketosis, where it primarily burns fat for fuel instead of carbohydrates, you can achieve remarkable results in weight management and health optimization.

However, starting a keto diet can be overwhelming, especially if you're unfamiliar with the principles and requirements of this unique dietary approach. That's where this ebook comes in. We have crafted this comprehensive guide to provide you with all the necessary information, guidance, and delicious recipes to embark on a successful ketogenic journey.

In the following pages, we will delve into the science behind the ketogenic diet and explore how it affects your body and metabolism. You'll gain a solid understanding of the macronutrient composition of a ketogenic diet, including the optimal ratios of fats, proteins, and carbohydrates, as well as the various types of ketogenic diets you can choose from.

We will also address common concerns and challenges beginners face, such as the dreaded "keto flu," dining out while on keto, and managing social situations. Additionally, we'll provide practical tips and strategies to help you stay motivated, maintain consistency, and overcome any obstacles that may arise along your ketogenic journey.

Of course, no guide to the ketogenic lifestyle would be complete without a collection of mouthwatering recipes. In this ebook, you'll find a diverse range of breakfast, lunch, dinner, snack, and dessert recipes, all carefully designed to be delicious, satisfying, and perfectly suited for beginners. Each recipe comes with detailed instructions, nutritional information, and helpful tips to ensure your success in the kitchen.

We've also included a sample meal plan to assist you in structuring your daily meals and making the transition to a keto diet smoother. This meal plan will provide you with a roadmap for incorporating the recipes into your routine and help you understand how to balance your macronutrient intake effectively.

Whether you're looking to shed excess weight, boost your energy levels, or improve your overall health, the ketogenic diet offers many benefits. With dedication, knowledge, and the right tools, you can unlock your body's potential to burn fat, achieve optimal health, and reach your weight loss goals.

So, without further ado, let's dive into the world of the ketogenic diet and begin your transformative journey towards a healthier, more vibrant you. Get ready to embrace the power of ketosis and discover the incredible array of delicious recipes in this "Keto Diet Cookbook For Beginners."

KETO RECIPES

BACON AND EGG BREAKFAST MUFFINS

Prep Time: 15 minutes Cooking Time: 20 minutes Servings: 6 muffins

Ingredients:

- Six slices of bacon
- Six large eggs
- 1/2 cup grated cheddar cheese
- 1/4 cup chopped green onions
- Salt and pepper, to taste
- Cooking spray or butter for greasing the muffin tin

Directions:

1. Preheat your oven to 375°F (190°C). Grease a 6-cup muffin tin with cooking spray or butter.

2. In a skillet over medium heat, cook the bacon until crispy. Remove the bacon from the skillet and place it on a paper towel to

drain excess grease. Once cooled, crumble the bacon into small pieces.

3. In a mixing bowl, crack the eggs and whisk them until well beaten. Add the grated cheddar cheese, chopped green onions, crumbled bacon, salt, and pepper. Mix everything until well combined.

4. Pour the egg mixture evenly into the prepared muffin tin, filling each cup about 3/4 full.

5. Place the muffin tin in the preheated oven and bake for approximately 15-20 minutes, or until the eggs are set, and the tops of the muffins are golden brown.

6. Once baked, remove the muffin tin from the oven and let the muffins cool for a few minutes. Use a knife or spatula to gently loosen the muffins from the tin, then transfer them to a wire rack to cool completely.

7. Serve the bacon and egg breakfast muffins warm or at room temperature. They can be enjoyed as is or paired with fresh fruit or a cup of coffee.

Nutrition Facts (per serving):

- Calories: 220

- Total Fat: 16g
- Saturated Fat: 7g
- Cholesterol: 230mg
- Sodium: 430mg
- Carbohydrates: 1g
- Protein: 17g

Note: The nutrition facts are approximate and may vary depending on the ingredients used.

AVOCADO EGG SALAD

Prep Time: 10 minutes Cooking Time: 10 minutes Serving: 4 servings

Ingredients:

- Four hard-boiled eggs, peeled and chopped
- Two ripe avocados, pitted and diced
- 1/4 cup red onion, finely chopped
- Two tablespoons fresh cilantro chopped
- One tablespoon of lime juice
- One tablespoon mayonnaise

- Salt and pepper to taste

Directions:

1. In a medium bowl, combine the chopped hard-boiled eggs, diced avocados, red onion, cilantro, lime juice, and mayonnaise.

2. Gently mix all the ingredients until well combined. Be careful not to mash the avocados completely, as some chunks will add texture to the salad.

3. Season with salt and pepper according to your taste preference.

4. Serve the avocado egg salad immediately or refrigerate for 30 minutes to allow the flavours to meld together.

5. Garnish with additional cilantro if desired.

6. Enjoy as a sandwich filling, on top of crackers, or as a salad on its own.

Nutrition Facts (per serving):

- Calories: 180
- Total Fat: 14g
- Saturated Fat: 2.5g
- Cholesterol: 186mg
- Sodium: 70mg
- Carbohydrates: 7g

- Fibre: 5g
- Sugar: 1g
- Protein: 7g
- Vitamin D: 0mcg
- Calcium: 28mg
- Iron: 1mg
- Potassium: 474mg

Please note that the nutrition facts are approximate and may vary depending on the specific ingredients and quantities used.

CAULIFLOWER FRIED RICE

Prep Time: 15 minutes Cooking Time: 15 minutes Serving: 4 servings

Ingredients:
- One medium-sized cauliflower
- Two tablespoons of vegetable oil
- One small onion, finely chopped
- Two cloves of garlic, minced
- One carrot, diced
- 1/2 cup frozen peas

- Two eggs, lightly beaten
- Two tablespoons of soy sauce
- One tablespoon of oyster sauce (optional)
- Salt and pepper to taste
- Green onions, chopped (for garnish)

Directions:

1. Cut the cauliflower into florets and remove the tough stems. Place the florets in a food processor and pulse until they resemble rice grains. Set aside.

2. Heat one tablespoon of vegetable oil in a large skillet or wok over medium heat. Add the chopped onion and minced garlic. Sauté for 2-3 minutes until the onion becomes translucent.

3. Add the diced carrot and frozen peas to the skillet. Stir-fry for another 2-3 minutes until the vegetables are tender.

4. Push the vegetables to one side of the skillet and pour the beaten eggs into the space. Scramble the eggs until cooked through.

5. Add the remaining tablespoon of vegetable oil to the skillet and add the cauliflower rice.

Stir-fry for 5-6 minutes until the cauliflower is tender but not mushy.

6. Pour the soy sauce and oyster sauce (if using) over the cauliflower rice. Stir to combine and evenly distribute the sauces. Cook for an additional 1-2 minutes to heat everything through.

7. Taste the cauliflower fried rice and season with salt and pepper according to your preference.

8. Remove from heat and garnish with chopped green onions.

Nutrition Facts (per serving):

- Calories: 120
- Total Fat: 6g
- Saturated Fat: 1g
- Cholesterol: 93mg
- Sodium: 560mg
- Total Carbohydrate: 12g
- Dietary Fiber: 4g
- Sugars: 5g
- Protein: 7g

Note: The nutrition facts may vary depending on the specific brands and quantities of ingredients used.

SPINACH AND FETA STUFFED CHICKEN BREAST

Prep Time: 20 minutes Cooking Time: 30 minutes Serving: 4 servings

Ingredients:

- Four boneless, skinless chicken breasts
- 1 cup fresh spinach, chopped
- 1/2 cup crumbled feta cheese
- Two cloves garlic, minced
- One teaspoon of dried oregano
- Salt and pepper, to taste
- One tablespoon of olive oil

Directions:

1. Preheat your oven to 375°F (190°C).

2. Butterfly the chicken breasts by slicing them horizontally, but not all the way through, so they can be opened like a book.

3. Mix the chopped spinach, feta cheese, minced garlic, dried oregano, salt, and pepper in a bowl.

4. Stuff each chicken breast with the spinach and feta mixture. Close the chicken breasts and secure them with toothpicks.

5. Heat the olive oil in an oven-safe skillet over medium-high heat. Once hot, add the stuffed chicken breasts and cook for 2-3 minutes on each side until browned.

6. Transfer the skillet with the chicken breasts to the preheated oven. Bake for about 20-25 minutes or until the chicken is cooked through and reaches an internal temperature of 165°F (74°C).

7. Remove the chicken breasts from the oven and let them rest for a few minutes. Remove the toothpicks before serving.

8. Serve the Spinach and Feta Stuffed Chicken Breast with your choice of side dishes like roasted vegetables, rice, or a salad.

Nutrition Facts (per serving):

- Calories: 250
- Fat: 10g
- Carbohydrates: 3g

- Protein: 35g
- Fibre: 1g

Note: The nutrition facts are approximate and may vary depending on the specific ingredients and serving size used.

ZUCCHINI NOODLES WITH CREAMY AVOCADO SAUCE

Prep Time: 15 minutes Cooking Time: 10 minutes Serving: 2

Ingredients:

- Two medium-sized zucchinis
- One ripe avocado
- 1/4 cup fresh basil leaves
- Two cloves of garlic, minced
- Two tablespoons of lemon juice
- Two tablespoons extra-virgin olive oil
- Salt and pepper to taste
- Optional toppings: cherry tomatoes, grated Parmesan cheese, chopped parsley

Directions:

1. Spiralize the zucchinis using a spiralizer or julienne peeler to create noodle-like strands. If you prefer softer noodles, lightly steam or blanch them for a minute and drain well.

2. In a blender or food processor, combine the ripe avocado, basil leaves, minced garlic, lemon juice, and extra-virgin olive oil. Blend until smooth and creamy. If the sauce is too thick, add a tablespoon of water until desired consistency is reached.

3. Heat a large skillet over medium heat and add a drizzle of olive oil. Add the zucchini noodles and sauté for about 3-4 minutes until they are tender but still slightly crunchy. Avoid overcooking as they can become mushy.

4. Pour the creamy avocado sauce over the zucchini noodles in the skillet. Toss gently to coat the noodles evenly with the sauce. Cook for another 1-2 minutes until the sauce is heated.

5. Season with salt and pepper to taste. If desired, add optional toppings such as halved cherry tomatoes, grated Parmesan

cheese, or chopped parsley for extra flavour and presentation.

6. Serve the zucchini noodles with creamy avocado sauce immediately as a main or side dish. Enjoy!

Nutrition Facts (per serving):

- Calories: 250
- Total Fat: 20g
- Saturated Fat: 3g
- Sodium: 150mg
- Total Carbohydrate: 17g
- Dietary Fiber: 10g
- Sugars: 4g
- Protein: 6g

Note: The nutrition facts are approximate and may vary based on the specific ingredients and quantities used.

KETO MEATBALLS WITH MARINARA SAUCE

Prep Time: 15 minutes Cooking Time: 25 minutes Serving: 4 servings

Ingredients: For the meatballs:

- 1 pound ground beef
- 1/4 cup almond flour
- 1/4 cup grated Parmesan cheese
- 1/4 cup chopped fresh parsley
- 1/4 cup minced onion
- One large egg
- Two cloves garlic, minced
- One teaspoon of dried oregano
- One teaspoon of dried basil
- 1/2 teaspoon salt
- 1/4 teaspoon black pepper

For the marinara sauce:

- One can (14 ounces) of crushed tomatoes
- Two tablespoons of tomato paste
- Two cloves garlic, minced
- 1/2 teaspoon dried basil
- 1/2 teaspoon dried oregano
- 1/4 teaspoon salt
- 1/4 teaspoon black pepper
- One tablespoon of olive oil

Directions:

1. Preheat your oven to 375°F (190°C).

2. In a large bowl, combine all the meatball ingredients. Mix well until everything is evenly combined.

3. Shape the mixture into golf ball-sized meatballs and place them on a baking sheet lined with parchment paper.

4. Bake the meatballs in the preheated oven for 20-25 minutes or until they are cooked through and browned.

5. While the meatballs are baking, prepare the marinara sauce. In a saucepan, heat the olive oil over medium heat. Add the minced garlic and cook for about 1 minute, until fragrant.

6. Stir in the crushed tomatoes, tomato paste, dried basil, dried oregano, salt, and black pepper. Simmer the sauce for 10-15 minutes, stirring occasionally.

7. Once the meatballs are cooked, transfer them to the saucepan with the marinara sauce. Gently stir to coat the meatballs with the sauce.

8. Allow the meatballs to simmer in the sauce for 5 minutes to soak up the flavours.

9. Serve the keto meatballs with hot marinara sauce, garnished with fresh parsley if desired.

Nutrition Facts (per serving):

- Calories: 330
- Total Fat: 21g
- Saturated Fat: 7g
- Cholesterol: 114mg
- Sodium: 663mg
- Total Carbohydrate: 9g
- Dietary Fiber: 3g
- Sugars: 4g
- Protein: 26g

Note: Nutrition facts are approximate and may vary depending on the specific ingredients and brands used.

GARLIC BUTTER SALMON

Prep Time: 10 minutes Cooking Time: 15 minutes Serving: 4 servings

Ingredients:

- Four salmon fillets
- Four tablespoons melted butter
- Four cloves garlic, minced
- Two tablespoons of fresh lemon juice
- One teaspoon of dried parsley
- Salt and pepper to taste
- Lemon wedges for serving
- Fresh parsley for garnish

Directions:

1. Preheat your oven to 400°F (200°C). Line a baking sheet with parchment paper or lightly grease it.

2. Place the salmon fillets on the prepared baking sheet.

3. In a small bowl, combine the melted butter, minced garlic, lemon juice, dried parsley, salt, and pepper. Stir well to make the garlic butter sauce.

4. Pour the garlic butter sauce over the salmon fillets, ensuring they are well coated.

5. Place the baking sheet in the preheated oven and bake for about 12-15 minutes, or until the salmon is cooked through and flakes easily with a fork.

6. Remove the salmon from the oven and let it rest for a few minutes.

7. Serve the Garlic Butter Salmon with lemon wedges on the side for squeezing over the fish. Garnish with fresh parsley.

Nutrition Facts (per serving):

- Calories: 300
- Total Fat: 18g
- Saturated Fat: 8g
- Cholesterol: 95mg
- Sodium: 150mg
- Carbohydrates: 1g
- Protein: 32g

Note: Nutrition facts may vary depending on the specific ingredients used and any modifications made to the recipe.

CHEESY CAULIFLOWER BREADSTICKS

Prep Time: 20 minutes Cooking Time: 30 minutes Serving: 4 servings

Ingredients:

- One medium cauliflower head

- Two large eggs
- 2 cups shredded mozzarella cheese
- 1/4 cup grated Parmesan cheese
- One teaspoon of dried oregano
- 1/2 teaspoon garlic powder
- 1/2 teaspoon salt
- 1/4 teaspoon black pepper
- Marinara sauce for serving

Directions:

1. Preheat your oven to 425°F (220°C). Line a baking sheet with parchment paper and set aside.

2. Cut the cauliflower head into florets, discarding the tough core. Place the florets in a food processor and pulse until they resemble rice-like grains.

3. Transfer the cauliflower "rice" to a microwave-safe bowl and microwave on high for 5 minutes, until tender. Allow it to cool for a few minutes.

4. Once the cauliflower has cooled, place it in a clean kitchen towel or cheesecloth. Squeeze out as much moisture as possible. This step is crucial to achieving a breadstick-like texture.

5. combine the squeezed cauliflower, eggs, shredded mozzarella cheese, grated Parmesan cheese, dried oregano, garlic powder, salt, and black pepper in a mixing bowl. Mix well until all the ingredients are thoroughly combined.

6. Transfer the mixture onto the prepared baking sheet. Using your hands, shape it into a rectangle or square about 1/2-inch thick.

7. Bake in the preheated oven for 25-30 minutes or until the edges are golden brown and the cheese is melted and bubbly.

8. Remove from the oven and let it cool for a few minutes. Using a sharp knife or pizza cutter, slice the cauliflower mixture into breadstick-sized pieces.

9. Serve the Cheesy Cauliflower Breadsticks warm with a marinara sauce for dipping.

Nutrition Facts (per serving):

- Calories: 180
- Fat: 11g
- Saturated Fat: 6g
- Cholesterol: 104mg
- Sodium: 496mg
- Carbohydrates: 6g

- Fibre: 2g
- Sugar: 3g
- Protein: 15g

Enjoy your Cheesy Cauliflower Breadsticks!

BROCCOLI AND CHEDDAR SOUP

Prep Time: 15 minutes Cooking Time: 30 minutes Serving: 4 servings

Ingredients:

- Two tablespoons butter
- One small onion, chopped
- Two cloves garlic, minced
- 4 cups broccoli florets
- 3 cups vegetable or chicken broth
- 1 cup milk
- 1 cup shredded cheddar cheese
- Salt and pepper to taste

Directions:

1. In a large pot, melt the butter over medium heat. Add the chopped onion and minced

garlic, and sauté until the onion becomes translucent about 5 minutes.

2. Add the broccoli florets to the pot and cook for another 5 minutes, stirring occasionally.

3. Pour in the vegetable or chicken broth and boil. Reduce the heat to low, cover the pot, and let the soup simmer for about 15 minutes or until the broccoli is tender.

4. Use an immersion blender or transfer the soup to a blender and blend until smooth. Be careful when blending hot liquids.

5. Return the blended soup to the pot (if using a blender) and stir in the milk. Heat the soup over medium-low heat until it is hot but not boiling.

6. Add the shredded cheddar cheese to the soup, stirring until it melts and incorporates into the soup.

7. Season with salt and pepper to taste. You can garnish the soup with additional shredded cheddar cheese or steamed broccoli florets if desired.

8. Serve the Broccoli and Cheddar Soup hot, and enjoy!

Nutrition Facts:

- Serving Size: 1 serving
- Calories: 280
- Total Fat: 18g
- Saturated Fat: 11g
- Cholesterol: 50mg
- Sodium: 800mg
- Total Carbohydrate: 18g
- Dietary Fiber: 4g
- Sugars: 7g
- Protein: 12g

Note: Nutrition facts may vary depending on the specific ingredients used and any modifications made to the recipe.

GREEK SALAD WITH GRILLED CHICKEN

Prep Time: 20 minutes Cooking Time: 15 minutes Serving: 4

Ingredients:

- Two boneless, skinless chicken breasts
- One tablespoon of olive oil

- One teaspoon of dried oregano
- Salt and pepper to taste
- 4 cups romaine lettuce, torn into bite-sized pieces
- 1 cup cherry tomatoes, halved
- One cucumber peeled, seeded, and diced
- 1/2 red onion, thinly sliced
- 1/2 cup Kalamata olives, pitted
- 1/2 cup crumbled feta cheese
- 1/4 cup fresh parsley, chopped

For the dressing:

- 1/4 cup extra-virgin olive oil
- Two tablespoons of red wine vinegar
- One clove of garlic, minced
- One teaspoon of dried oregano
- Salt and pepper to taste

Directions:

1. Preheat your grill to medium-high heat. Season the chicken breasts with olive oil, dried oregano, salt, and pepper. Grill the chicken for about 6-8 minutes per side or until cooked through. Remove from the grill

and let it rest for a few minutes. Slice the chicken into thin strips.

2. In a large bowl, combine the romaine lettuce, cherry tomatoes, cucumber, red onion, Kalamata olives, crumbled feta cheese, and chopped parsley.

3. In a small bowl, whisk together the extra-virgin olive oil, red wine vinegar, minced garlic, dried oregano, salt, and pepper to make the dressing.

4. Pour the dressing over the salad ingredients and toss well to coat.

5. Divide the salad among four plates and top each portion with the grilled chicken strips.

6. Serve immediately and enjoy!

Nutrition Facts (per serving): Calories: 320 Total Fat: 20g Saturated Fat: 6g Cholesterol: 75mg Sodium: 600mg Total Carbohydrate: 10g Dietary Fiber: 3g Sugars: 5g Protein: 25g

Note: Nutrition facts are approximate and may vary depending on the ingredients used.

BACON-WRAPPED ASPARAGUS

Prep Time: 15 minutes Cooking Time: 20 minutes Serving: 4 servings

Ingredients:

- One bunch of asparagus spears (about 1 pound)
- 8 slices of bacon
- Olive oil (for drizzling)
- Salt and pepper (to taste)

Directions:

1. Preheat your oven to 400°F (200°C). Line a baking sheet with parchment paper or aluminium foil for easy cleanup.

2. Trim the tough ends of the asparagus spears about 1-2 inches from the bottom.

3. Divide the asparagus into eight equal bundles. Take a slice of bacon and wrap it tightly around each bundle, starting from the bottom and working your way up.

4. Place the bacon-wrapped asparagus bundles on the prepared baking sheet, seam side down. Drizzle a little olive oil over each bundle and season with salt and pepper to taste.

5. Bake in the oven for about 20 minutes or until the bacon is crispy and the asparagus is

tender. You can broil for the last 1-2 minutes to make the bacon extra crispy if desired.

6. Remove from the oven and let them cool for a few minutes. Serve the bacon-wrapped asparagus as a side dish or as an appetizer.

Nutrition Facts (per serving):

- Calories: 160
- Fat: 11g
- Cholesterol: 25mg
- Sodium: 410mg
- Carbohydrates: 5g
- Fibre: 2g
- Protein: 9g

Note: The nutrition facts are approximate and may vary depending on the specific ingredients and quantities used.

COCONUT CURRY CHICKEN

Prep Time: 15 minutes Cooking Time: 30 minutes Serving: 4

Ingredients:

- 1.5 lbs (680g) boneless, skinless chicken breasts cut into bite-sized pieces
- One tablespoon of vegetable oil
- One onion, finely chopped
- Three cloves garlic, minced
- 1 tablespoon grated fresh ginger
- Two tablespoons of curry powder
- One teaspoon of ground cumin
- 1 teaspoon ground coriander
- 1/2 teaspoon turmeric powder
- One can (13.5 oz/400ml) of coconut milk
- 1 cup chicken broth
- Two tablespoons of soy sauce
- One tablespoon of brown sugar
- One tablespoon of fish sauce
- Juice of 1 lime
- Fresh cilantro leaves for garnish
- Cooked rice for serving

Directions:

1. heat the vegetable oil over medium heat in a large skillet or wok. Add the chopped onion and cook until it becomes translucent about

3-4 minutes. Stir in the minced garlic and grated ginger, and cook for another minute.

2. In a small bowl, combine the curry powder, ground cumin, ground coriander, and turmeric powder. Add the spice mixture to the skillet and cook, stirring constantly, for about 1 minute to toast the spices.

3. Push the onion and spice mixture to one side of the skillet and add the chicken pieces to the other. Cook the chicken until it is browned on all sides, about 5-6 minutes.

4. Pour in the coconut milk, chicken broth, soy sauce, brown sugar, and fish sauce. Stir well to combine all the ingredients. Bring the mixture to a simmer, reduce the heat to low, cover the skillet, and let it cook for about 15-20 minutes or until the chicken is cooked through and tender.

5. Stir in the lime juice and cook for 2 minutes. Taste and adjust the seasoning if needed.

6. Serve the coconut curry chicken over cooked rice. Garnish with fresh cilantro leaves.

Nutrition Facts (per serving):

- Calories: 360

- Total Fat: 18g
- Saturated Fat: 12g
- Cholesterol: 96mg
- Sodium: 810mg
- Carbohydrates: 11g
- Fibre: 2g
- Sugar: 4g
- Protein: 38g

Note: Nutrition facts may vary depending on the specific ingredients and brands used.

PORTOBELLO MUSHROOM PIZZAS

Prep Time: 15 minutes Cooking Time: 20 minutes Servings: 4

Ingredients:

- Four large Portobello mushrooms
- 1 cup pizza sauce
- 1 cup shredded mozzarella cheese
- 1/4 cup sliced black olives
- 1/4 cup sliced cherry tomatoes
- 1/4 cup sliced fresh basil leaves

- Salt and pepper to taste
- Olive oil for brushing

Directions:

1. Preheat your oven to 375°F (190°C). Line a baking sheet with parchment paper.

2. Clean the Portobello mushrooms by gently wiping them with a damp cloth. Remove the stems and gills from the mushrooms.

3. Place the mushrooms on the prepared baking sheet and gill side up. Brush the mushroom caps with olive oil and season with salt and pepper.

4. Spread about two tablespoons of pizza sauce on each mushroom cap.

5. Sprinkle shredded mozzarella cheese evenly over the sauce.

6. Top the pizzas with sliced black olives, cherry tomatoes, and fresh basil leaves.

7. Bake in the preheated oven for about 15-20 minutes or until the mushrooms are tender and the cheese is melted and bubbly.

8. Remove from the oven and let them cool for a few minutes before serving.

9. Serve the Portobello Mushroom Pizzas hot as an appetizer or a main dish.

Nutrition Facts: (Per Serving) Calories: 120 Total Fat: 7g Saturated Fat: 3g Cholesterol: 15mg Sodium: 300mg Total Carbohydrate: 8g Dietary Fiber: 2g Sugars: 4g Protein: 7g

Note: The nutrition facts are approximate and may vary depending on the ingredients used.

SAUSAGE AND EGG BREAKFAST CASSEROLE

Prep Time: 20 minutes Cooking Time: 45 minutes Serving: 6-8 servings

Ingredients:

- 1 pound breakfast sausage
- Six slices of bread cubed
- 1 1/2 cups shredded cheddar cheese
- Six large eggs
- 2 cups milk
- One teaspoon mustard
- 1/2 teaspoon salt
- 1/4 teaspoon black pepper
- 1/4 teaspoon garlic powder

- 1/4 teaspoon onion powder
- 1/4 teaspoon paprika
- Fresh parsley, chopped (for garnish)

Directions:

1. Preheat your oven to 350°F (175°C). Grease a 9x13-inch baking dish.

2. In a large skillet, cook the breakfast sausage over medium heat until browned and cooked through. Remove from heat and drain any excess grease.

3. Place the cubed bread in the prepared baking dish. Sprinkle the cooked sausage evenly over the bread cubes. Top with shredded cheddar cheese.

4. In a medium bowl, whisk together the eggs, milk, mustard, salt, black pepper, garlic powder, onion powder, and paprika until well combined.

5. Pour the egg mixture evenly over the bread, sausage, and cheese in the baking dish. Press down on the ingredients with a spatula to ensure they are fully submerged in the egg mixture.

6. Cover the baking dish with aluminium foil and bake in the oven for 30 minutes.

7. After 30 minutes, remove the foil and continue baking for another 10-15 minutes or until the casserole is set and the top is golden brown.

8. Once cooked, remove the casserole from the oven and let it cool for a few minutes. Garnish with chopped fresh parsley.

9. Slice the casserole into squares and serve warm. Enjoy!

Nutrition Facts (per serving):

- Calories: 380
- Fat: 25g
- Saturated Fat: 10g
- Cholesterol: 230mg
- Sodium: 790mg
- Carbohydrates: 17g
- Fibre: 1g
- Sugar: 4g
- Protein: 20g

Please note that these nutrition facts are approximate and may vary depending on the ingredients and brands used.

LEMON GARLIC SHRIMP SKEWERS

Prep Time: 15 minutes Cooking Time: 10 minutes Serving: 4 servings

Ingredients:

- 1 pound large shrimp, peeled and deveined
- Three cloves garlic, minced
- Two tablespoons of fresh lemon juice
- Two tablespoons of olive oil
- One teaspoon of lemon zest
- 1/2 teaspoon salt
- 1/4 teaspoon black pepper
- 1/4 teaspoon red pepper flakes (optional)
- Wooden skewers, soaked in water for 30 minutes

Directions:

1. In a bowl, combine the minced garlic, lemon juice, olive oil, lemon zest, salt, black pepper, and red pepper flakes (if using). Mix well.

2. Add the peeled and deveined shrimp to the bowl and toss to coat them evenly with the marinade. Let it marinate for about 10 minutes.

3. Preheat the grill to medium-high heat.

4. Thread the marinated shrimp onto the soaked wooden skewers, piercing them through the tail and head sections.

5. Place the shrimp skewers on the preheated grill and cook for about 3-4 minutes per side or until the shrimp turn pink and opaque.

6. Remove the skewers from the grill and transfer them to a serving plate.

7. Serve the lemon garlic shrimp skewers hot as an appetizer or main course. You can squeeze some additional lemon juice over the top if desired.

Nutrition Facts (per serving):

- Calories: 180
- Total Fat: 8g
- Saturated Fat: 1g
- Cholesterol: 220mg
- Sodium: 480mg
- Carbohydrates: 2g

- Fibre: 0g
- Sugar: 0g
- Protein: 24g

Note: The nutrition facts provided are approximate and may vary depending on the specific ingredients and quantities used.

KETO TACO SALAD

Prep Time: 15 minutes Cooking Time: 15 minutes Serving: 4

Ingredients:

- 1 pound ground beef
- One tablespoon of taco seasoning (look for a low-carb version or make your own)
- 4 cups lettuce (romaine or iceberg), chopped
- 1 cup cherry tomatoes, halved
- One avocado, diced
- 1/2 cup shredded cheddar cheese
- 1/4 cup sliced black olives
- 1/4 cup diced red onion

- 1/4 cup chopped fresh cilantro
- 1/4 cup sour cream
- 2 tablespoons salsa
- One tablespoon of lime juice
- Salt and pepper to taste

Directions:

1. In a large skillet, cook the ground beef over medium heat until browned. Drain any excess fat.

2. Sprinkle the taco seasoning over the ground beef and stir well to coat. Cook for an additional 2-3 minutes to allow the flavours to meld. Remove from heat and set aside.

3. In a large bowl, combine the lettuce, cherry tomatoes, avocado, cheddar cheese, black olives, red onion, and cilantro.

4. In a small bowl, whisk together the sour cream, salsa, lime juice, salt, and pepper to make the dressing.

5. Add the cooked ground beef to the bowl of salad ingredients and toss everything together.

6. Drizzle the dressing over the salad and toss again to ensure everything is coated.

7. Serve the Keto Taco Salad in individual bowls or plates.

8. You can garnish with additional cilantro and a squeeze of lime juice if desired.

Nutrition Facts (per serving):

- Calories: 380
- Fat: 27g
- Carbohydrates: 10g
- Fibre: 7g
- Protein: 26g

Note: Nutrition facts may vary depending on the specific ingredients and brands used.

CHEESY BACON BRUSSELS SPROUTS

Prep Time: 15 minutes Cooking Time: 25 minutes Serving: 4

Ingredients:

- 1 pound Brussels sprouts, trimmed and halved
- Four slices bacon, cooked and crumbled
- 1 cup shredded cheddar cheese
- 1/4 cup grated Parmesan cheese

- 1/4 cup breadcrumbs
- Two tablespoons butter, melted
- 1/2 teaspoon garlic powder
- Salt and pepper to taste

Directions:

1. Preheat your oven to 400°F (200°C). Grease a baking dish with cooking spray or butter and set aside.

2. Bring a large pot of salted water to a boil. Add the Brussels sprouts and cook for about 5 minutes until they are slightly tender. Drain and set aside.

3. In a mixing bowl, combine the cooked and crumbled bacon, cheddar cheese, Parmesan cheese, breadcrumbs, melted butter, garlic powder, salt, and pepper. Mix well until all the ingredients are evenly incorporated.

4. Place the blanched Brussels sprouts in the greased baking dish. Sprinkle the bacon and cheese mixture evenly over the top.

5. Place the baking dish in the preheated oven and bake for about 20 minutes, or until the cheese is melted and bubbly and the Brussels sprouts are cooked through.

6. Once done, remove it from the oven and let it cool for a few minutes. Serve the Cheesy Bacon Brussels Sprouts as a delicious side dish to accompany your main course.

Nutrition Facts (per serving):

- Calories: 240
- Total Fat: 17g
- Saturated Fat: 9g
- Cholesterol: 45mg
- Sodium: 400mg
- Total Carbohydrate: 11g
- Dietary Fiber: 4g
- Sugars: 2g
- Protein: 13g

Note: Nutritional values may vary depending on the specific brands of ingredients used and any modifications made to the recipe.

BUFFALO CHICKEN LETTUCE WRAPS

Prep Time: 15 minutes Cooking Time: 15 minutes Servings: 4

Ingredients:

- 1 pound boneless, skinless chicken breasts, cooked and shredded
- 1/2 cup buffalo sauce
- 1/4 cup ranch dressing
- 1/4 cup chopped green onions
- 1/4 cup crumbled blue cheese
- Eight large lettuce leaves (such as romaine or iceberg)
- Optional toppings: diced tomatoes, sliced avocado, chopped cilantro

Directions:

1. In a large bowl, combine the shredded chicken and buffalo sauce. Mix well until the chicken is evenly coated.

2. Heat a skillet over medium heat and add the buffalo chicken mixture. Cook for 5-7 minutes, stirring occasionally, until heated through.

3. While the chicken is cooking, prepare the lettuce leaves by washing and drying them thoroughly. Trim off any excess stems.

4. Once the chicken is cooked, remove it from the heat and let it cool slightly.

5. To assemble the lettuce wraps, take a leaf and spoon a portion of the buffalo chicken mixture onto the centre of the leaf.

6. Drizzle some ranch dressing over the chicken and sprinkle with green onions and blue cheese.

7. Add any optional toppings you desire, such as diced tomatoes, sliced avocado, or chopped cilantro.

8. Fold the sides of the lettuce leaf over the filling, then roll it up tightly to form a wrap. Repeat with the remaining ingredients.

9. Serve the buffalo chicken lettuce wraps immediately as a light and flavorful meal or as an appetizer.

Nutrition Facts: Serving Size: 1 lettuce wrap Calories: 180 Total Fat: 8g

- Saturated Fat: 2g
- Trans Fat: 0g Cholesterol: 55mg Sodium: 680mg Total Carbohydrate: 4g
- Dietary Fiber: 1g
- Sugars: 2g Protein: 23g

Note: Nutrition facts may vary depending on the brand of buffalo sauce, ranch dressing, and blue cheese used. Optional toppings are not included in the provided nutrition information.

CAULIFLOWER MAC AND CHEESE

Prep Time: 15 minutes Cooking Time: 35 minutes Serving: 4 servings

Ingredients:

- One medium-sized cauliflower head
- 8 ounces of elbow macaroni
- 2 cups shredded cheddar cheese
- 1 cup milk
- Two tablespoons unsalted butter
- Two tablespoons all-purpose flour
- 1/2 teaspoon garlic powder
- 1/2 teaspoon onion powder
- 1/4 teaspoon paprika
- Salt and pepper to taste
- Fresh parsley (optional, for garnish)

Directions:

1. Preheat your oven to 375°F (190°C). Grease a 9x13-inch baking dish and set aside.

2. Cut the cauliflower head into small florets and discard the tough stem. Rinse the florets under cold water and set aside.

3. Bring a large pot of salted water to a boil. Cook the elbow macaroni according to the package instructions until al dente. Drain the cooked macaroni and set aside.

4. In a separate saucepan, melt the butter over medium heat. Add the flour and whisk continuously for 1-2 minutes until the mixture is smooth and bubbling.

5. Slowly pour in the milk while whisking constantly to prevent lumps from forming. Continue cooking and whisking until the mixture thickens and comes to a simmer.

6. Add the garlic powder, onion powder, paprika, salt, and pepper to the sauce, and stir until well combined.

7. Remove the saucepan from the heat, and gradually add the shredded cheddar cheese while stirring constantly until melted and smooth.

8. In a large mixing bowl, combine the cooked macaroni, cauliflower florets, and cheese sauce. Toss gently until the macaroni and cauliflower are evenly coated.

9. Transfer the mixture to the greased baking dish, spreading it out evenly.

10. Bake in the preheated oven for 20-25 minutes or until the top is golden brown and bubbling.

11. Remove from the oven and let it cool for a few minutes. Garnish with fresh parsley if desired.

12. Serve the cauliflower mac and cheese while it's still warm, and enjoy!

Nutrition Facts (per serving):

- Calories: 350
- Fat: 18g
- Saturated Fat: 10g
- Cholesterol: 50mg
- Sodium: 350mg
- Carbohydrates: 30g
- Fibre: 3g
- Sugar: 5g
- Protein: 17g

Note: The nutrition facts are approximate and may vary depending on the specific ingredients and quantities used.

CAPRESE STUFFED AVOCADO

Prep Time: 10 minutes Cooking Time: 0 minutes Serving: 2 servings

Ingredients:

- Two ripe avocados
- 1 cup cherry tomatoes, halved
- 8 ounces fresh mozzarella cheese, cubed
- 1/4 cup fresh basil leaves, chopped
- Two tablespoons balsamic glaze
- Salt and pepper, to taste

Directions:

1. Cut the avocados in half lengthwise and remove the pits. Scoop out a bit of flesh from each avocado half to create a larger cavity.

2. In a bowl, combine the cherry tomatoes, mozzarella cheese, and chopped basil leaves. Mix well.

3. Season the tomato and cheese mixture with salt and pepper to taste.

4. Fill each avocado half with the tomato and cheese mixture, pressing gently to fill the cavity.

5. Drizzle each stuffed avocado with balsamic glaze.

6. Serve the Caprese stuffed avocados immediately and enjoy!

Nutrition Facts: (Per serving) Calories: 320 Fat: 24g Saturated Fat: 8g Cholesterol: 35mg Sodium: 290mg Carbohydrates: 15g Fiber: 9g Sugar: 4g Protein: 14g Vitamin D: 0mcg Calcium: 300mg Iron: 1mg Potassium: 790mg

KETO CHICKEN PARMESAN

Prep Time: 15 minutes Cooking Time: 30 minutes Serving: 4 servings

Ingredients:

- Four boneless, skinless chicken breasts
- 1 cup almond flour
- 1/2 cup grated Parmesan cheese
- One teaspoon garlic powder
- One teaspoon dried oregano
- One teaspoon dried basil
- 1/2 teaspoon salt

- 1/4 teaspoon black pepper
- Two large eggs, beaten
- 1 cup sugar-free marinara sauce
- 1 cup shredded mozzarella cheese
- Fresh basil leaves, for garnish (optional)

Directions:

1. Preheat your oven to 400°F (200°C) and line a baking sheet with parchment paper.

2. In a shallow bowl, combine the almond flour, grated Parmesan cheese, garlic powder, dried oregano, dried basil, salt, and black pepper.

3. Dip each chicken breast into the beaten eggs, then coat it evenly with the almond flour mixture. Place the coated chicken breasts on the prepared baking sheet.

4. Bake the chicken breasts in the preheated oven for about 20 minutes or until they are cooked through and golden brown.

5. Remove the chicken from the oven and spoon marinara sauce over each chicken breast. Sprinkle shredded mozzarella cheese on top.

6. Return the chicken to the oven and bake for an additional 10 minutes or until the cheese is melted and bubbly.

7. Once cooked, remove the chicken from the oven and let it rest for a few minutes.

8. Serve the Keto Chicken Parmesan with additional marinara sauce if desired, and garnish with fresh basil leaves if you like. Enjoy!

Nutrition Facts (per serving):

- Calories: 350
- Fat: 20g
- Protein: 35g
- Carbohydrates: 7g
- Fibre: 3g
- Net Carbs: 4g

CHEESY GARLIC ROASTED BROCCOLI

Prep Time: 10 minutes Cooking Time: 20 minutes Serving: 4

Ingredients:

- One large head of broccoli, cut into florets
- Two tablespoons olive oil
- Three cloves of garlic, minced
- 1/2 teaspoon salt
- 1/4 teaspoon black pepper
- 1/2 cup grated cheddar cheese

Directions:

1. Preheat the oven to 425°F (220°C).

2. In a large bowl, combine the broccoli florets, olive oil, minced garlic, salt, and black pepper. Toss well to ensure the broccoli is evenly coated with the mixture.

3. Spread the broccoli in a single layer on a baking sheet lined with parchment paper or aluminium foil.

4. Roast the broccoli in the preheated oven for about 15-20 minutes or until the florets are tender and slightly crispy around the edges.

5. Remove the baking sheet from the oven and sprinkle the grated cheddar cheese evenly over the roasted broccoli.

6. Return the baking sheet to the oven for an additional 2-3 minutes or until the cheese has melted and started to bubble.

7. Carefully remove the baking sheet from the oven and let the cheesy garlic roasted broccoli cool for a few minutes before serving.

Nutrition Facts:

- Serving Size: 1/4 of the recipe
- Calories: 150
- Total Fat: 10g
- Saturated Fat: 3g
- Cholesterol: 10mg
- Sodium: 400mg
- Total Carbohydrate: 12g
- Dietary Fiber: 5g
- Sugars: 3g
- Protein: 7g

Enjoy your delicious cheesy garlic-roasted broccoli!

SPINACH AND MUSHROOM STUFFED PORK TENDERLOIN

Prep Time: 20 minutes Cooking Time: 40 minutes Serving: 4 servings

Ingredients:

- One pork tenderloin (about 1.5 pounds)
- 2 cups fresh spinach leaves
- 1 cup sliced mushrooms
- Two cloves garlic, minced
- 1/4 cup grated Parmesan cheese
- 1/4 cup bread crumbs
- One tablespoon olive oil
- One teaspoon dried thyme
- 1/2 teaspoon salt
- 1/4 teaspoon black pepper
- Cooking twine or toothpicks

Directions:

1. Preheat the oven to 375°F (190°C).

2. Butterfly the pork tenderloin by making a lengthwise cut down the centre, without cutting all the way through, so that you can open it like a book.

3. In a skillet, heat the olive oil over medium heat. Add the garlic and sauté for 1 minute until fragrant.

4. Add the mushrooms to the skillet and cook for 4-5 minutes until they release their moisture and start to brown.

5. Stir in the spinach leaves and cook until wilted. Remove the skillet from heat and let the mixture cool slightly.

6. In a bowl, combine the Parmesan cheese, bread crumbs, dried thyme, salt, and black pepper.

7. Spread the spinach and mushroom mixture evenly over the opened pork tenderloin.

8. Sprinkle the breadcrumb mixture over the spinach and mushroom layer.

9. Carefully roll the pork tenderloin, starting from one end, to enclose the filling. Secure the roll with cooking twine or toothpicks.

10. Place the stuffed pork tenderloin in a baking dish and roast in the preheated oven for 30-35 minutes or until the internal temperature reaches 145°F (63°C).

11. Remove the pork tenderloin from the oven and let it rest for 5 minutes before slicing.

12. Remove the cooking twine or toothpicks and slice the pork tenderloin into rounds.

13. Serve the Spinach and Mushroom Stuffed Pork Tenderloin with your favourite sides or a fresh salad.

Nutrition Facts (per serving):

- Calories: 310
- Fat: 13g
- Protein: 38g
- Carbohydrates: 7g
- Fibre: 2g

Note: Nutrition facts may vary depending on the specific ingredients and quantities used.

BACON-WRAPPED JALAPENO POPPERS

Prep Time: 20 minutes Cooking Time: 20 minutes Serving: 12 poppers

Ingredients:

- 12 jalapeno peppers

- Six slices of bacon
- 4 ounces cream cheese, softened
- 1/2 cup shredded cheddar cheese
- 1/2 teaspoon garlic powder
- 1/2 teaspoon onion powder
- 1/4 teaspoon paprika
- Salt and pepper to taste
- Toothpicks

Directions:

1. Preheat your oven to 375°F (190°C) and line a baking sheet with aluminium foil.

2. Cut each jalapeno pepper in half lengthwise. Remove the seeds and membranes using a small spoon or knife. Wear gloves to protect your hands from the jalapeno's heat.

3. In a bowl, combine the softened cream cheese, shredded cheddar cheese, garlic powder, onion powder, paprika, salt, and pepper. Mix well until all the ingredients are evenly incorporated.

4. Fill each jalapeno half with the cream cheese mixture, using a spoon or your fingers to press it firmly into the cavity.

5. Take a slice of bacon and cut it in half widthwise. Wrap each stuffed jalapeno half with a half slice of bacon, securing it with a toothpick to hold it in place.

6. Arrange the bacon-wrapped jalapeno poppers on the prepared baking sheet, leaving some space between each one.

7. Place the baking sheet in the oven and bake for about 20 minutes or until the bacon is crispy and the jalapenos are tender.

8. Once cooked, remove the toothpicks from the poppers and let them cool for a few minutes before serving.

9. Serve the Bacon-Wrapped Jalapeno Poppers as an appetizer or party snack. Enjoy!

Nutrition Facts (per serving): Calories: 124 Total Fat: 10g

- Saturated Fat: 5g
- Trans Fat: 0g Cholesterol: 27mg Sodium: 216mg Total Carbohydrate: 2g
- Dietary Fiber: 0g
- Sugars: 1g Protein: 6g

Please note that the nutrition facts may vary depending on the specific brands and quantities of ingredients used.

CREAMY TUSCAN GARLIC CHICKEN

Prep Time: 15 minutes Cooking Time: 20 minutes Serving: 4 servings

Ingredients:

- Four boneless, skinless chicken breasts
- Salt and pepper, to taste
- Two tablespoons olive oil
- Four cloves garlic, minced
- 1 cup cherry tomatoes, halved
- 1 cup baby spinach
- 1 cup heavy cream
- ½ cup grated Parmesan cheese
- One teaspoon dried Italian seasoning
- Fresh basil leaves for garnish

Directions:

1. Season the chicken breasts with salt and pepper on both sides.

2. Heat olive oil in a large skillet over medium-high heat. Add the chicken breasts and cook for about 6-7 minutes per side or until browned and cooked. Remove the chicken from the skillet and set aside.

3. In the same skillet, add the minced garlic and sauté for about 1 minute until fragrant.

4. Add the cherry tomatoes and cook for another 2-3 minutes until they soften.

5. Stir in the baby spinach and cook until wilted.

6. Reduce the heat to low and pour in the heavy cream. Stir in the Parmesan cheese and dried Italian seasoning. Simmer for about 2-3 minutes until the sauce thickens slightly.

7. Return the chicken breasts to the skillet, coating them with creamy sauce. Cook for an additional 2-3 minutes until the chicken is heated through.

8. Garnish with fresh basil leaves before serving.

Nutrition Facts (per serving):

- Calories: 420
- Fat: 28g

- Carbohydrates: 6g
- Protein: 35g
- Fibre: 1g

Note: The nutrition facts are approximate and may vary depending on the ingredients used.

BAKED ZUCCHINI FRIES

Prep Time: 15 minutes Cooking Time: 25 minutes Serving: 4 servings

Ingredients:

- Two medium zucchini
- 1/2 cup all-purpose flour
- Two large eggs, beaten
- 1 cup breadcrumbs
- 1/4 cup grated Parmesan cheese
- One teaspoon garlic powder
- 1/2 teaspoon paprika
- 1/2 teaspoon salt
- 1/4 teaspoon black pepper
- Cooking spray

Directions:

1. Preheat your oven to 425°F (220°C). Line a baking sheet with parchment paper and set aside.

2. Wash the zucchini and cut off the ends. Cut the zucchini into fry-shaped pieces, about 1/2 inch wide and 3 inches long.

3. In three separate bowls, set up your breading station. In the first bowl, place the flour. In the second bowl, beat the eggs. In the third bowl, combine the breadcrumbs, grated Parmesan cheese, garlic powder, paprika, salt, and black pepper.

4. Take each zucchini piece and dip it first in the flour, shaking off any excess. Then dip it into the beaten eggs, allowing any excess to drip off. Finally, coat the zucchini piece in the breadcrumb mixture, pressing gently to adhere the crumbs.

5. Place the breaded zucchini fries on the prepared baking sheet, leaving space between each fry. Lightly spray the fries with cooking spray to help them crisp up.

6. Bake in the preheated oven for about 20-25 minutes or until the fries are golden brown

and crispy. Flip the fries halfway through the baking time to ensure even browning.

7. Once done, remove the fries from the oven and let them cool for a few minutes. Serve the baked zucchini fries hot with your favourite dipping sauce.

Nutrition Facts (per serving):

- Calories: 170
- Fat: 4g
- Saturated Fat: 1.5g
- Cholesterol: 82mg
- Sodium: 485mg
- Carbohydrates: 25g
- Fibre: 2g
- Sugar: 3g
- Protein: 9g
- Vitamin A: 6%
- Vitamin C: 35%
- Calcium: 12%
- Iron: 12%

STEAK WITH BLUE CHEESE BUTTER

Prep Time: 10 minutes Cooking Time: 15 minutes Serving: 2 servings

Ingredients:

- Two ribeye or sirloin steaks (approximately 1 inch thick)
- Salt and pepper, to taste
- Two tablespoons olive oil
- Four tablespoons unsalted butter, softened
- 2 ounces blue cheese, crumbled
- Two tablespoons fresh parsley, chopped
- One garlic clove, minced

Directions:

1. Preheat a grill or grill pan over medium-high heat.

2. Season the steaks generously with salt and pepper on both sides.

3. Drizzle the olive oil over the steaks and rub it in to coat them evenly.

4. Place the steaks on the preheated grill or grill pan and cook for about 4-5 minutes per side for medium-rare, or adjust the cooking

time according to your desired level of doneness.

5. While the steaks are cooking, prepare the blue cheese butter. Combine the softened butter, crumbled blue cheese, chopped parsley, and minced garlic in a small bowl. Mix well until all the ingredients are evenly incorporated.

6. Once the steaks are done, remove them from the grill and let them rest for a few minutes.

7. While the steaks are resting, place a dollop of the blue cheese butter on top of each steak. Allow the butter to melt and spread over the surface of the steak.

8. Serve the steak with your choice of sides, such as roasted potatoes or a fresh salad.

Nutrition Facts (per serving):

- Calories: 450
- Total Fat: 36g
- Saturated Fat: 16g
- Cholesterol: 120mg
- Sodium: 450mg
- Protein: 30g
- Carbohydrate: 1g

- Fibre: 0g
- Sugar: 0g

Note: The nutrition facts provided are approximate and may vary depending on the specific ingredients used and the serving size.

MEXICAN CAULIFLOWER RICE

Prep Time: 10 minutes Cooking Time: 15 minutes Serving: 4 servings

Ingredients:
- One medium cauliflower head
- One tablespoon olive oil
- One small onion, finely diced
- Two cloves garlic, minced
- One red bell pepper, diced
- One jalapeno pepper, seeded and finely diced
- One teaspoon ground cumin
- One teaspoon chili powder
- 1/2 teaspoon paprika
- Salt and pepper to taste

- 1/4 cup chopped fresh cilantro
- Juice of 1 lime

Directions:

1. Remove the leaves and core of the cauliflower head. Cut the cauliflower into florets, then pulse them in a food processor until they resemble rice grains.

2. Heat the olive oil in a large skillet or frying pan over medium heat. Add the diced onion, minced garlic, and sauté until they become fragrant and translucent for about 2-3 minutes.

3. Add the diced red bell pepper and jalapeno pepper to the skillet, and cook for another 2-3 minutes until they soften.

4. Add the cauliflower rice to the skillet, stirring well to combine with the other ingredients. Cook for about 5 minutes, until the cauliflower rice is tender but still slightly crisp.

5. Mix the ground cumin, chilli powder, paprika, salt, and pepper in a small bowl. Sprinkle this spice mixture over the cauliflower rice, and stir well to coat evenly.

6. Continue cooking for another 2-3 minutes, allowing the spices to blend and the flavours to develop.

7. Remove the skillet from the heat. Stir in the chopped cilantro and squeeze the lime juice over the cauliflower rice. Toss everything together until well combined.

8. Serve the Mexican Cauliflower Rice as a side dish with your favourite Mexican-inspired main course, or use it as a filling for tacos or burritos.

Nutrition Facts (per serving):

- Calories: 80
- Total Fat: 4g
- Saturated Fat: 0.5g
- Cholesterol: 0mg
- Sodium: 110mg
- Total Carbohydrate: 9g
- Dietary Fiber: 3g
- Sugars: 4g
- Protein: 3g

Note: The nutrition facts are approximate and may vary depending on the specific ingredients and brands used.

EGGPLANT PARMESAN

Prep Time: 30 minutes Cooking Time: 45 minutes Serving: 4 servings

Ingredients:

- Two large eggplants
- 2 cups breadcrumbs
- 1 cup all-purpose flour
- Four eggs, beaten
- 2 cups marinara sauce
- 2 cups shredded mozzarella cheese
- 1 cup grated Parmesan cheese
- 1/4 cup fresh basil leaves, chopped
- 1/4 cup fresh parsley leaves, chopped
- Salt and pepper, to taste
- Olive oil for frying

Directions:

1. Preheat the oven to 375°F (190°C).

2. Slice the eggplants into 1/4-inch thick rounds. Place them in a colander and sprinkle salt over them. Let them sit for about 15 minutes to release excess moisture.

Rinse the slices and pat them dry with a paper towel.

3. Set up a breading station with three shallow bowls. In the first bowl, place the flour. In the second bowl, beat the eggs. In the third bowl, place the breadcrumbs.

4. Dip each eggplant slice into the flour, shaking off any excess. Then dip it into the beaten eggs, allowing any excess to drip off. Finally, coat it with breadcrumbs, pressing gently to adhere. Repeat with the remaining slices.

5. Heat olive oil in a large skillet over medium-high heat. Fry the breaded eggplant slices in batches until golden brown on both sides, about 3-4 minutes per side. Place the cooked slices on a paper towel-lined plate to absorb any excess oil.

GARLIC BUTTER SHRIMP AND BROCCOLI

Prep Time: 10 minutes Cooking Time: 15 minutes Serving: 4

Ingredients:

- 1 pound (450g) shrimp, peeled and deveined
- 3 cups broccoli florets
- Four tablespoons butter
- Four cloves garlic, minced
- One teaspoon paprika
- Salt and black pepper, to taste
- Fresh parsley, chopped (for garnish)
- Lemon wedges (for serving)

Directions:

1. In a large pot of salted boiling water, blanch the broccoli florets for 2-3 minutes until tender. Drain and set aside.

2. In a large skillet, melt the butter over medium heat. Add the minced garlic and cook for 1-2 minutes until fragrant.

3. Add the shrimp to the skillet and season with paprika, salt, and black pepper. Cook for

3-4 minutes, stirring occasionally, until the shrimp turn pink and opaque.

4. Add the blanched broccoli florets to the skillet and toss with the garlic butter shrimp. Cook for 2-3 minutes to heat through and allow the flavours to combine.

5. Remove from heat and garnish with fresh chopped parsley.

6. Serve the garlic butter shrimp and broccoli hot with lemon wedges on the side for squeezing over the dish.

Nutrition Facts (per serving):

- Calories: 240
- Total Fat: 12g
- Saturated Fat: 7g
- Cholesterol: 190mg
- Sodium: 360mg
- Carbohydrates: 7g
- Fibre: 3g
- Sugar: 2g
- Protein: 26g

Note: Nutrition facts are approximate and may vary depending on the ingredients used.

KETO PIZZA CASSEROLE

Prep Time: 15 minutes Cooking Time: 35 minutes Serving: 6 servings

Ingredients:

- 1 pound ground beef
- One medium onion, diced
- Two cloves garlic, minced
- 1 cup low-sugar marinara sauce
- One teaspoon of dried oregano
- One teaspoon of dried basil
- 1/2 teaspoon salt
- 1/4 teaspoon black pepper
- 2 cups shredded mozzarella cheese
- 1/4 cup sliced black olives
- 1/4 cup sliced pepperoni
- Fresh basil leaves, for garnish (optional)

Directions:

1. Preheat your oven to 375°F (190°C). Grease a 9x13-inch baking dish.

2. In a large skillet, cook the ground beef over medium heat until browned. Drain the excess fat.

3. Add the diced onion and minced garlic to the skillet with the ground beef. Cook for 2-3 minutes until the onion becomes translucent.

4. Stir in the marinara sauce, dried oregano, dried basil, salt, and black pepper. Simmer the mixture for 5 minutes, allowing the flavours to blend.

5. Spread half of the meat sauce evenly into the prepared baking dish.

6. Sprinkle half of the shredded mozzarella cheese over the meat sauce.

7. Layer the remaining meat sauce on top, followed by the remaining mozzarella cheese.

8. Arrange the sliced black olives and pepperoni on top of the casserole.

9. Bake in the preheated oven for 25-30 minutes or until the cheese is melted and bubbly.

10. Once done, remove from the oven and let it cool for a few minutes.

11. Garnish with fresh basil leaves, if desired, before serving.

Nutrition Facts (per serving):

- Calories: 320
- Total Fat: 23g
- Saturated Fat: 10g
- Cholesterol: 78mg
- Sodium: 640mg
- Total Carbohydrate: 5g
- Dietary Fiber: 1g
- Sugars: 2g
- Protein: 24g

Note: Nutrition facts are approximate and may vary depending on the ingredients used.

Enjoy your delicious Keto Pizza Casserole!

GREEK CHICKEN SKEWERS WITH TZATZIKI SAUCE

Prep Time: 15 minutes Cooking Time: 15 minutes Serving: 4 servings

Ingredients:

- 1.5 pounds boneless, skinless chicken breasts cut into 1-inch cubes
- 1/4 cup extra-virgin olive oil

- Three tablespoons freshly squeezed lemon juice
- Two teaspoons of dried oregano
- Two cloves garlic, minced
- Salt and black pepper, to taste
- One large cucumber, peeled and grated
- 1 cup Greek yoghurt
- Two tablespoons of freshly squeezed lemon juice
- Two cloves garlic, minced
- One tablespoon of chopped fresh dill
- Salt and black pepper, to taste
- Wooden skewers, soaked in water for 30 minutes

Directions:

1. In a large bowl, combine the olive oil, lemon juice, dried oregano, minced garlic, salt, and black pepper. Add the chicken cubes to the bowl and toss until well coated. Marinate the chicken in the refrigerator for at least 1 hour or overnight for best results.

2. In the meantime, prepare the tzatziki sauce. Place the grated cucumber in a fine-mesh sieve or colander and squeeze out any

excess moisture. Combine the grated cucumber, Greek yoghurt, lemon juice, minced garlic, chopped dill, salt, and black pepper in a medium bowl. Stir well to combine. Cover the bowl and refrigerate the tzatziki sauce until ready to serve.

3. Preheat your grill or grill pan over medium-high heat. Thread the marinated chicken cubes onto the soaked wooden skewers, dividing them evenly.

4. Place the chicken skewers on the grill and cook for about 6-8 minutes per side, or until the chicken is cooked through and has a nice charred exterior.

5. Once cooked, remove the chicken skewers from the grill and let them rest for a few minutes.

6. Serve the Greek chicken skewers with the tzatziki sauce on the side. If desired, you can also serve them with warm pita bread, sliced tomatoes, red onions, and fresh herbs.

Nutrition Facts (per serving):

- Calories: 320
- Total Fat: 12g
- Saturated Fat: 2g

- Cholesterol: 95mg
- Sodium: 220mg
- Total Carbohydrate: 6g
- Dietary Fiber: 1g
- Sugars: 3g
- Protein: 44g

Enjoy your delicious Greek Chicken Skewers with Tzatziki Sauce!

BACON AND CHEESE STUFFED BELL PEPPERS

Prep Time: 20 minutes Cooking Time: 35 minutes Serving: 4 servings

Ingredients:

- Four large bell peppers (any colour)
- Eight slices of bacon
- One small onion, finely chopped
- Two cloves of garlic, minced
- 1 cup shredded cheddar cheese
- 1 cup cooked rice
- 1/2 teaspoon dried oregano

- 1/2 teaspoon dried basil
- Salt and pepper to taste
- Fresh parsley, chopped (for garnish)

Directions:

1. Preheat your oven to 375°F (190°C).

2. Cut off the tops of the bell peppers and remove the seeds and membranes from the inside. Rinse them thoroughly.

3. In a skillet, cook the bacon over medium heat until crispy. Remove the bacon from the skillet and drain on paper towels. Once cooled, crumble the bacon into small pieces.

4. In the same skillet, using the bacon fat, sauté the chopped onion and minced garlic until they become soft and translucent.

5. In a large bowl, combine the crumbled bacon, cooked onion and garlic mixture, shredded cheddar cheese, cooked rice, dried oregano, dried basil, salt, and pepper. Mix well until all the ingredients are evenly distributed.

6. Stuff the bell peppers with the bacon and cheese mixture, pressing it down firmly to fill them.

7. Place the stuffed bell peppers in a baking dish and cover with aluminium foil.

8. Bake in the preheated oven for 25 minutes. Then, remove the foil and bake for an additional 10 minutes, or until the bell peppers are tender and the cheese is melted and bubbly.

9. Once cooked, remove the stuffed bell peppers from the oven and let them cool for a few minutes.

10. Garnish with freshly chopped parsley before serving. Enjoy your delicious bacon and cheese stuffed bell peppers!

Nutrition Facts (per serving):

- Calories: 320
- Total Fat: 18g
- Saturated Fat: 8g
- Cholesterol: 45mg
- Sodium: 560mg
- Total Carbohydrate: 25g
- Dietary Fiber: 3g
- Sugars: 6g
- Protein: 15g

Please note that the nutrition facts are approximate and may vary based on the specific ingredients and brands used.

LEMON HERB ROASTED CHICKEN THIGHS

Prep Time: 10 minutes Cooking Time: 35 minutes Serving: 4 servings

Ingredients:

- Eight chicken thighs, bone-in and skin-on
- Two lemons, juiced and zested
- 3 cloves of garlic, minced
- Two tablespoons fresh thyme leaves chopped
- Two tablespoons fresh rosemary leaves, chopped
- Two tablespoons of olive oil
- Salt and black pepper, to taste

Directions:

1. Preheat your oven to 400°F (200°C).

2. In a small bowl, combine the lemon juice, lemon zest, minced garlic, thyme, rosemary, olive oil, salt, and black pepper. Mix well.

3. Place the chicken thighs in a large mixing bowl and pour the lemon herb mixture. Toss the chicken thighs to coat them evenly with the mixture.

4. Transfer the chicken thighs to a baking dish, arranging them in a single layer with the skin side up.

5. Pour any remaining marinade over the chicken thighs.

6. Place the baking dish in the preheated oven and roast for about 35 minutes or until the chicken thighs are cooked through, and the skin is golden brown and crispy.

7. Once cooked, remove the chicken thighs from the oven and let them rest for a few minutes before serving.

8. Serve the Lemon Herb Roasted Chicken Thighs hot and garnish with additional lemon slices, if desired.

Nutrition Facts (per serving):

- Calories: 350
- Fat: 24g

- Carbohydrates: 3g
- Protein: 30g
- Fibre: 1g

Note: The nutrition facts provided are estimates and may vary based on the specific ingredients used.

CABBAGE AND SAUSAGE STIR-FRY

Prep Time: 10 minutes Cooking Time: 15 minutes Serving: 4 servings

Ingredients:

- One medium cabbage, thinly sliced
- Four sausages (your choice of flavour), sliced
- One onion, thinly sliced
- Two cloves of garlic, minced
- One red bell pepper, thinly sliced
- Two tablespoons of soy sauce
- One tablespoon of oyster sauce
- One teaspoon of sesame oil
- 1/2 teaspoon red pepper flakes (optional)

- Salt and pepper to taste
- Two tablespoons of cooking oil

Directions:

1. Heat one tablespoon of cooking oil in a large skillet or wok over medium-high heat.

2. Add the sliced sausages until they are browned and cooked through. Remove them from the skillet and set aside.

3. In the same skillet, add another tablespoon of cooking oil and sauté the minced garlic and sliced onion until they become fragrant and slightly translucent.

4. Add the sliced cabbage and red bell pepper to the skillet and stir-fry for about 5-7 minutes until the cabbage starts to wilt.

5. Return the cooked sausages to the skillet and mix them with the vegetables.

6. In a small bowl, whisk together the soy sauce, oyster sauce, sesame oil, red pepper flakes (if using), salt, and pepper.

7. Pour the sauce mixture over the cabbage and sausage in the skillet and stir-fry for 2-3 minutes until everything is well coated and heated.

8. Taste and adjust the seasoning if needed.

9. Remove from heat and serve the cabbage and sausage stir-fry hot with steamed rice or noodles.

Nutrition Facts (per serving):

- Calories: 320
- Fat: 23g
- Carbohydrates: 15g
- Protein: 13g
- Fibre: 5g
- Sugar: 8g
- Sodium: 900mg

Note: Nutrition facts may vary depending on the type and brand of sausages used.

ZUCCHINI LASAGNA

Prep Time: 20 minutes Cooking Time: 1 hour Serving: 6 servings

Ingredients:

- Four medium zucchinis
- One tablespoon of olive oil
- One onion, chopped
- Three cloves garlic, minced

- 1 pound ground beef (or substitute with ground turkey or vegetarian ground meat)
- One can (14 ounces) of crushed tomatoes
- One can (6 ounces) of tomato paste
- One teaspoon of dried basil
- One teaspoon of dried oregano
- 1/2 teaspoon salt
- 1/4 teaspoon black pepper
- 2 cups ricotta cheese
- One egg
- 2 cups shredded mozzarella cheese
- 1/2 cup grated Parmesan cheese
- Fresh basil leaves, for garnish (optional)

Directions:

1. Preheat your oven to 375°F (190°C). Grease a 9x13-inch baking dish with cooking spray and set it aside.

2. Slice the zucchinis lengthwise into thin strips, about 1/4-inch thick. You can use a mandoline or a sharp knife to achieve even slices. Lay the zucchini slices on paper towels and sprinkle them with salt. Let them sit for

about 10 minutes to release excess moisture, then pat them dry with paper towels.

3. heat the olive oil over medium heat in a large skillet. Add the chopped onion, minced garlic, and sauté until they become fragrant, and the onion turns translucent, about 3-4 minutes.

4. Add the ground beef to the skillet and cook, breaking it up with a spoon, until it is browned and cooked through. Drain any excess fat from the skillet.

5. Stir in the crushed tomatoes, tomato paste, dried basil, dried oregano, salt, and black pepper. Simmer the sauce for about 10 minutes to allow the flavours to meld together.

6. In a small bowl, combine the ricotta cheese and egg. Mix well until smooth and set aside.

7. To assemble the lasagna, spread a thin layer of the meat sauce on the bottom of the prepared baking dish. Arrange a single layer of zucchini slices on top. Spread half of the ricotta cheese mixture evenly over the zucchini, followed by a layer of the meat sauce. Sprinkle a third of the mozzarella cheese and Parmesan cheese on top.

8. Repeat the layers with the remaining zucchini slices, ricotta cheese mixture, meat sauce, and another third of the mozzarella and Parmesan cheese.

9. For the final layer, arrange the zucchini slices on top and cover them with the remaining meat sauce. Sprinkle the remaining mozzarella and Parmesan cheese over the sauce.

10. Cover the baking dish with foil and bake in the oven for 40 minutes. Then, remove the foil and bake for 15-20 minutes or until the cheese is golden and bubbly.

11. Once done, remove the lasagna from the oven and let it cool for a few minutes. Garnish with fresh basil leaves, if desired, before serving.

Nutrition Facts (per serving): Calories: 365 Total Fat: 21g

- Saturated Fat: 10g
- Trans Fat: 0g Cholesterol: 106mg Sodium: 684mg Total Carbohydrate: 13g
- Dietary Fiber: 3g
- Sugars: 7g Protein: 30g

Note: Nutritional values are approximate and may vary depending on the ingredients used.

CREAMY GARLIC PARMESAN MUSHROOMS

Prep Time: 10 minutes Cooking Time: 15 minutes Serving: 4 servings

Ingredients:

- 1 lb (450g) mushrooms, sliced
- Two tablespoons butter
- Four cloves garlic, minced
- 1 cup heavy cream
- 1/2 cup grated Parmesan cheese
- Salt and pepper to taste
- Fresh parsley, chopped (for garnish)

Directions:

1. In a large skillet, melt the butter over medium heat.

2. Add the minced garlic and sauté for about 1 minute until fragrant.

3. Add the sliced mushrooms to the skillet and cook for 5-7 minutes, stirring occasionally, until they have released their moisture and are tender.

4. Reduce the heat to low and pour in the heavy cream. Stir well to combine.

5. Sprinkle in the grated Parmesan cheese and continue stirring until the cheese has melted and the sauce is smooth and creamy. This should take about 3-4 minutes.

6. Season with salt and pepper to taste. Taste the sauce before adding too much salt, as Parmesan cheese can be salty.

7. Remove from heat and garnish with freshly chopped parsley.

8. Serve the creamy garlic Parmesan mushrooms as a side dish or overcooked pasta, rice, or crusty bread for a delicious main course.

Nutrition Facts (per serving):

- Calories: 230
- Fat: 19g
- Saturated Fat: 12g
- Cholesterol: 65mg
- Sodium: 300mg

- Carbohydrates: 7g
- Fibre: 1g
- Sugar: 2g
- Protein: 8g

Note: The nutrition facts provided are approximate and may vary based on the specific ingredients used and the serving size.

BBQ PULLED PORK LETTUCE WRAPS

Prep Time: 15 minutes Cooking Time: 6 hours Servings: 4

Ingredients:

- 2 pounds of pork shoulder or pork butt
- 1 cup barbecue sauce
- 1/2 cup chicken broth
- Two tablespoons brown sugar
- Two tablespoons of apple cider vinegar
- One tablespoon of Worcestershire sauce
- One teaspoon of smoked paprika
- 1/2 teaspoon garlic powder

- 1/2 teaspoon onion powder
- Salt and pepper, to taste
- Eight large lettuce leaves (such as iceberg or butter lettuce)
- Optional toppings: diced tomatoes, shredded cheese, sliced red onions, chopped cilantro

Directions:

1. In a slow cooker, combine the barbecue sauce, chicken broth, brown sugar, apple cider vinegar, Worcestershire sauce, smoked paprika, garlic powder, onion powder, salt, and pepper. Stir well to combine.

2. Add the pork shoulder or pork butt to the slow cooker and coat it with the barbecue sauce mixture.

3. Cover the slow cooker and cook on low heat for 6 hours or until the pork is tender and easily shreds with a fork.

4. Once the pork is cooked, remove it from the slow cooker and shred it using two forks.

5. Return the shredded pork to the slow cooker and stir it in the sauce to coat evenly. Cook for an additional 30 minutes on low heat.

6. To serve, spoon the BBQ-pulled pork onto lettuce leaves. Top with optional toppings such as diced tomatoes, shredded cheese, sliced red onions, and chopped cilantro.

7. Roll up the lettuce leaves like a wrap, tucking in the sides as you go.

Nutrition Facts (per serving):

- Calories: 450
- Fat: 20g
- Carbohydrates: 30g
- Protein: 35g
- Fibre: 2g
- Sugar: 23g
- Sodium: 800mg

Enjoy your delicious BBQ Pulled Pork Lettuce Wraps!

CHEESY BACON CAULIFLOWER CASSEROLE

Prep Time: 15 minutes Cooking Time: 45 minutes Serving: 6 servings

Ingredients:

- One large head of cauliflower, cut into florets
- Six slices of bacon, cooked and crumbled
- 1 cup shredded cheddar cheese
- 1 cup shredded mozzarella cheese
- 1/2 cup grated Parmesan cheese
- 1/2 cup sour cream
- 1/2 cup mayonnaise
- 2 cloves garlic, minced
- 1/2 teaspoon dried thyme
- 1/2 teaspoon dried oregano
- Salt and pepper to taste
- Chopped fresh parsley for garnish (optional)

Directions:

1. Preheat your oven to 375°F (190°C). Grease a 9x13-inch baking dish and set aside.

2. Fill a large pot with water and bring it to a boil. Add the cauliflower florets and cook for 5 minutes or until they are tender-crisp. Drain the cauliflower and set aside.

3. In a large mixing bowl, combine the cooked bacon, cheddar cheese, mozzarella

cheese, Parmesan cheese, sour cream, mayonnaise, minced garlic, dried thyme, dried oregano, salt, and pepper. Mix well until all the ingredients are evenly combined.

4. Add the cooked cauliflower to the cheese and bacon mixture. Gently toss until the cauliflower is coated with the mixture.

5. Transfer the mixture to the greased baking dish and spread it out evenly.

6. Bake in the oven for 25-30 minutes or until the casserole is golden brown and bubbly.

7. Remove from the oven and let it cool for a few minutes. Garnish with chopped fresh parsley, if desired.

8. Serve the Cheesy Bacon Cauliflower Casserole hot, and enjoy!

Nutrition Facts (per serving):

- Calories: 280
- Total Fat: 23g
- Saturated Fat: 10g
- Cholesterol: 52mg
- Sodium: 530mg
- Total Carbohydrate: 7g

- Dietary Fiber: 2g
- Sugars: 3g
- Protein: 12g

Note: The nutrition facts provided are estimates and may vary based on the specific ingredients used.

GRILLED LEMON HERB PORK CHOPS

Prep Time: 15 minutes Cooking Time: 10 minutes Serving: 4

Ingredients:

- Four boneless pork chops, about 1 inch thick
- Two lemons
- Three tablespoons olive oil
- Two cloves garlic, minced
- One tablespoon of fresh rosemary, chopped
- One tablespoon of fresh thyme, chopped
- Salt and pepper to taste

Directions:

1. Preheat the grill to medium-high heat.

2. Squeeze the juice of one lemon into a small bowl. Add the olive oil, minced garlic, rosemary, thyme, salt, and pepper. Stir well to combine.

3. Place the pork chops in a shallow dish and pour the lemon herb marinade over them. Make sure the pork chops are evenly coated. Allow them to marinate for 10 minutes, turning them once or twice to ensure even flavour distribution.

4. While the pork chops are marinating, cut the remaining lemon into thin slices.

5. Once the grill is hot, remove the pork chops from the marinade and shake off any excess. Discard the remaining marinade.

6. Place the pork chops on the grill and cook for about 4-5 minutes per side or until they reach an internal temperature of 145°F (63°C). Cooking time may vary depending on the thickness of the chops.

7. During the last few minutes of cooking, place the lemon slices on the grill and cook until they have grill marks and have softened slightly.

8. Once the pork chops are cooked, remove them from the grill and let them rest for a couple of minutes. This allows the juices to redistribute and keeps them tender.

9. Serve the grilled lemon herb pork chops with the grilled lemon slices on top. You can squeeze some of the grilled lemon juice over the chops for an extra flavour.

Nutrition Facts (per serving):

- Calories: 280
- Total Fat: 16g
- Saturated Fat: 3g
- Cholesterol: 75mg
- Sodium: 70mg
- Carbohydrates: 5g
- Fibre: 1g
- Sugar: 1g
- Protein: 28g

Note: The nutrition facts are approximate and may vary depending on the specific ingredients used and portion sizes.

STUFFED PORTOBELLO MUSHROOMS WITH SPINACH AND CHEESE

Prep Time: 20 minutes Cooking Time: 25 minutes Serving: 4

Ingredients:

- Four large Portobello mushrooms
- Two tablespoons olive oil
- Two cloves garlic, minced
- One small onion, finely chopped
- 2 cups fresh spinach, chopped
- 1 cup shredded mozzarella cheese
- 1/4 cup grated Parmesan cheese
- Salt and pepper to taste

Directions:

1. Preheat the oven to 375°F (190°C). Line a baking sheet with parchment paper.

2. Clean the Portobello mushrooms by removing the stems and gently wiping the caps with a damp cloth. Place them on the prepared baking sheet, gill-side up.

3. In a skillet, heat the olive oil over medium heat. Add the minced garlic and chopped onion. Sauté for 2-3 minutes until the onion becomes translucent.

4. Add the chopped spinach to the skillet and cook until wilted about 2 minutes. Remove from heat.

5. In a bowl, combine the sautéed spinach mixture, shredded mozzarella cheese, grated Parmesan cheese, salt, and pepper. Mix well.

6. Spoon the spinach and cheese mixture into each Portobello mushroom cap, dividing it evenly among the mushrooms. Press it down gently to fill the caps.

7. Bake the stuffed mushrooms in the preheated oven for 20-25 minutes, or until the mushrooms are tender and the cheese is melted and golden brown on top.

8. Remove from the oven and let them cool for a few minutes before serving.

9. Serve the stuffed Portobello mushrooms as a delicious appetizer or side dish. Enjoy!

Nutrition Facts (per serving):

- Calories: 170
- Fat: 11g
- Carbohydrates: 9g
- Fibre: 2g
- Protein: 10g
- Sodium: 250mg

Note: The nutrition facts are approximate and may vary depending on the specific ingredients and brands used.

KETO-FRIENDLY BEEF STROGANOFF

Prep Time: 10 minutes Cooking Time: 30 minutes Serving: 4 servings

Ingredients:

- 1.5 pounds (680g) beef sirloin, thinly sliced
- Two tablespoons of olive oil
- One medium onion, thinly sliced
- Three cloves garlic, minced
- 8 ounces (225g) mushrooms, sliced
- 1 cup beef broth
- One tablespoon of Worcestershire sauce
- One teaspoon of Dijon mustard
- 1/2 cup sour cream
- Salt and pepper to taste
- Fresh parsley, chopped (for garnish)

Directions:

1. Heat the olive oil in a large skillet over medium-high heat. Add the sliced beef and cook until browned, about 2-3 minutes per side. Remove the beef from the skillet and set aside.

2. add the sliced onions and minced garlic in the same skillet. Sauté until the onions are translucent and fragrant, about 3-4 minutes.

3. Add the sliced mushrooms to the skillet and cook until they have softened and released their moisture, about 5 minutes.

4. Return the beef to the skillet and stir in the beef broth, Worcestershire sauce, and Dijon mustard. Season with salt and pepper to taste. Bring the mixture to a simmer and let it cook for 10-15 minutes, allowing the flavours to meld together.

5. Reduce the heat to low and stir in the sour cream. Cook for an additional 2-3 minutes, stirring constantly, until the sauce has thickened slightly.

6. Remove from heat and garnish with fresh chopped parsley.

7. Serve the Keto-friendly Beef Stroganoff hot over cauliflower rice or zucchini noodles.

Nutrition Facts (per serving):

- Calories: 345
- Fat: 22g
- Carbohydrates: 6g
- Fibre: 1g
- Protein: 30g

Note: The nutrition facts are approximate and may vary depending on the ingredients used.

BAKED PARMESAN ZUCCHINI CHIPS

Prep Time: 15 minutes Cooking Time: 20 minutes Serving: 4 servings

Ingredients:

- Two medium zucchinis
- 1/2 cup grated Parmesan cheese
- 1/2 cup breadcrumbs
- 1/2 teaspoon garlic powder
- 1/2 teaspoon paprika
- 1/4 teaspoon salt
- 1/4 teaspoon black pepper
- Two large eggs

Directions:

1. Preheat your oven to 425°F (220°C). Line a baking sheet with parchment paper or lightly grease it.

2. Wash the zucchinis and slice them into thin rounds, about 1/4 inch thick. Pat them dry with a paper towel to remove excess moisture.

3. In a shallow bowl, whisk the eggs until well beaten.

4. In another bowl, combine the grated Parmesan cheese, breadcrumbs, garlic powder, paprika, salt, and black pepper. Mix well.

5. Dip each zucchini round into the beaten eggs, coating both sides. Then, press each side of the zucchini round into the Parmesan mixture, ensuring it's fully coated. Place the coated zucchini round onto the prepared baking sheet. Repeat the process with the remaining zucchini rounds.

6. Bake the zucchini chips in the oven for about 10 minutes. Carefully flip the chips over and bake for an additional 10 minutes or until they turn golden brown and crispy.

7. Once cooked, remove the baking sheet from the oven and let the zucchini chips cool for a few minutes before serving.

8. Serve the Baked Parmesan Zucchini Chips as a tasty snack or a side dish with your favourite dipping sauce.

Nutrition Facts (per serving):

- Calories: 138
- Fat: 7g
- Carbohydrates: 12g
- Fibre: 2g
- Protein: 9g
- Sugar: 2g
- Sodium: 482mg

Note: The nutrition facts are approximate and may vary depending on the specific ingredients and brands used.

CHICKEN CAESAR SALAD WRAPS

Prep Time: 15 minutes Cooking Time: 10 minutes Serving: 4

Ingredients:

- 2 cups cooked chicken breast, shredded
- 1/2 cup Caesar salad dressing
- 1/4 cup grated Parmesan cheese
- 1/4 cup chopped fresh parsley
- Four large flour tortillas
- 2 cups romaine lettuce, chopped
- 1/2 cup cherry tomatoes, halved
- 1/4 cup sliced black olives (optional)
- Salt and pepper to taste

Directions:

1. In a mixing bowl, combine the shredded chicken, Caesar salad dressing, Parmesan cheese, and chopped parsley. Mix well until the chicken is coated with the dressing.

2. Lay out the flour tortillas on a clean surface. Divide the chicken mixture equally among the tortillas and spread it out in the centre.

3. Top the chicken with chopped romaine lettuce, cherry tomatoes, and sliced black olives (if desired). Sprinkle with salt and pepper to taste.

4. Fold the sides of the tortillas inward, then roll them up tightly to form wraps.

5. If desired, you can secure the wraps with toothpicks to hold them together.

6. Serve the Chicken Caesar Salad Wraps immediately, or you can wrap them in plastic wrap and refrigerate them for later. They are great for packed lunches or picnics!

Nutrition Facts: The following nutrition facts are approximate and may vary depending on the specific ingredients used.

Serving Size: 1 wrap Calories: 380 Total Fat: 18g

- Saturated Fat: 5g
- Trans Fat: 0g Cholesterol: 70mg Sodium: 800mg Total Carbohydrate: 28g
- Dietary Fiber: 3g
- Sugars: 2g Protein: 27g

Note: The nutrition facts provided are estimates and may vary based on the specific ingredients and brands used in the recipe.

CREAMY GARLIC BUTTER TUSCAN SHRIMP

Prep Time: 10 minutes Cooking Time: 20 minutes Serving: 4 servings

Ingredients:

- 1 pound (450g) shrimp, peeled and deveined
- Two tablespoons butter
- Four cloves garlic, minced
- One small onion, finely chopped
- 1 cup cherry tomatoes, halved
- 1 cup baby spinach leaves
- 1 cup heavy cream
- 1/2 cup grated Parmesan cheese
- 1/2 teaspoon dried basil
- 1/2 teaspoon dried oregano
- Salt and black pepper to taste
- Fresh parsley, chopped (for garnish)

Directions:

1. In a large skillet, melt the butter over medium heat. Add the minced garlic, chopped onion, and sauté until fragrant and onions are translucent.

2. Add the shrimp to the skillet and cook for 2-3 minutes per side until they turn pink and

opaque. Remove the shrimp from the skillet and set aside.

3. In the same skillet, add the halved cherry tomatoes and cook for 2-3 minutes until they soften.

4. Stir in the baby spinach leaves and cook until wilted.

5. Reduce the heat to low and pour in the heavy cream. Stir in the grated Parmesan cheese, dried basil, dried oregano, salt, and black pepper. Cook for 2-3 minutes, until the sauce thickens slightly.

6. Return the cooked shrimp to the skillet and toss them in the creamy sauce until well-coated. Cook for an additional 2-3 minutes to heat the shrimp through.

7. Remove from heat and garnish with freshly chopped parsley.

8. Serve the Creamy Garlic Butter Tuscan Shrimp over cooked pasta or with crusty bread.

Nutrition Facts (per serving):

- Calories: 410
- Fat: 28g
- Saturated Fat: 17g

- Cholesterol: 286mg
- Sodium: 615mg
- Carbohydrates: 8g
- Fibre: 1g
- Sugar: 3g
- Protein: 33g

Enjoy your Creamy Garlic Butter Tuscan Shrimp!

CABBAGE ROLL CASSEROLE

Prep Time: 20 minutes Cooking Time: 1 hour Serving: 6 servings

Ingredients:

- One large head of cabbage
- 1 pound ground beef
- One onion, finely chopped
- Two cloves of garlic, minced
- 1 cup cooked rice
- One can (14 ounces) of diced tomatoes
- One can (8 ounces) of tomato sauce
- One tablespoon of tomato paste

- 1 teaspoon dried oregano
- One teaspoon of dried basil
- 1/2 teaspoon paprika
- 1/2 teaspoon salt
- 1/4 teaspoon black pepper
- 1 cup shredded mozzarella cheese
- Fresh parsley, chopped (for garnish)

Directions:

1. Preheat your oven to 350°F (175°C).

2. Fill a large pot with water and bring it to a boil. Carefully remove the outer leaves of the cabbage, discarding any damaged leaves. Place the cabbage head in the boiling water and cook for about 5-7 minutes or until the leaves are tender and pliable. Remove the cabbage from the water and set it aside to cool.

3. In a large skillet, cook the ground beef over medium heat until browned. Add the chopped onion and minced garlic to the skillet and cook until the onion is translucent.

4. Stir in the cooked rice, diced tomatoes, tomato sauce, tomato paste, dried oregano, dried basil, paprika, salt, and black pepper.

Simmer the mixture for 5-7 minutes, allowing the flavours to blend.

5. Grease a casserole dish with non-stick cooking spray. Take a cabbage leaf and place a spoonful of the meat and rice mixture onto the centre of the leaf. Roll the leaf tightly, tucking in the sides as you go, and place it seam-side down in the prepared casserole dish. Repeat this process with the remaining cabbage leaves and filling until all the ingredients are used.

6. Pour any remaining sauce over the cabbage rolls in the casserole dish. Cover the dish with foil and bake in the preheated oven for 45 minutes.

7. After 45 minutes, remove the foil and sprinkle the shredded mozzarella cheese over the top of the casserole. Return the dish to the oven and bake uncovered for 10-15 minutes or until the cheese is melted and bubbly.

8. Remove the cabbage roll casserole from the oven and let it cool for a few minutes. Garnish with freshly chopped parsley before serving.

Nutrition Facts (per serving):

- Calories: 340
- Total Fat: 18g
- Saturated Fat: 8g
- Cholesterol: 65mg
- Sodium: 760mg
- Total Carbohydrate: 23g
- Dietary Fiber: 5g
- Sugars: 9g
- Protein: 22g

Note: The nutrition information is an estimate and may vary depending on the ingredients used.

SAUSAGE AND SPINACH STUFFED MUSHROOMS

Prep Time: 15 minutes Cooking Time: 25 minutes Servings: 4

Ingredients:

- 24 large mushrooms, stems removed
- 1/2 pound Italian sausage, casings removed
- 2 cups fresh spinach, chopped

- 1/2 cup breadcrumbs
- 1/4 cup grated Parmesan cheese
- Two cloves garlic, minced
- 1/4 teaspoon dried oregano
- 1/4 teaspoon dried basil
- Salt and pepper to taste
- Two tablespoons of olive oil

Directions:

1. Preheat the oven to 375°F (190°C). Line a baking sheet with parchment paper.

2. In a large skillet, cook the Italian sausage over medium heat, breaking it into small pieces with a spoon until browned and cooked through. Remove the sausage from the skillet and set aside.

3. In the same skillet, add the chopped spinach and cook until wilted, about 2-3 minutes. Remove the spinach from the skillet and set aside.

4. In a bowl, combine the cooked sausage, spinach, breadcrumbs, Parmesan cheese, minced garlic, dried oregano, dried basil, salt, and pepper. Mix well until all the ingredients are evenly combined.

5. Stuff each mushroom cap with a spoonful of the sausage and spinach mixture, pressing it down lightly.

6. Arrange the stuffed mushrooms on the prepared baking sheet. Drizzle olive oil over the mushrooms.

7. Bake in the preheated oven for 20-25 minutes or until the mushrooms are tender and the stuffing is golden brown.

8. Remove from the oven and let cool for a few minutes before serving.

9. Serve the sausage and spinach stuffed mushrooms as an appetizer or side dish.

Nutrition Facts (per serving): Calories: 243 Fat: 16g Saturated Fat: 5g Cholesterol: 30mg Sodium: 538mg Carbohydrates: 16g Fiber: 3g Sugar: 3g Protein: 10g

Note: Nutrition facts are approximate and may vary depending on the ingredients used.

LEMON DILL SALMON WITH CUCUMBER SALAD

Prep Time: 15 minutes Cooking Time: 15 minutes Serving: 4

Ingredients:

- Four salmon fillets
- Two lemons divided
- Two tablespoons fresh dill chopped
- Salt and pepper, to taste
- Two cucumbers, thinly sliced
- 1/2 red onion, thinly sliced
- Two tablespoons fresh parsley chopped
- Two tablespoons of olive oil
- One tablespoon of white vinegar

Directions:

1. Preheat your oven to 400°F (200°C). Line a baking sheet with parchment paper.

2. Place the salmon fillets on the prepared baking sheet. Squeeze the juice of one lemon over the salmon. Sprinkle with fresh dill, salt, and pepper.

3. Bake the salmon in the preheated oven for about 12-15 minutes or until it flakes easily with a fork.

4. While the salmon is baking, prepare the cucumber salad. In a bowl, combine the

sliced cucumbers, red onion, and fresh parsley.

5. In a small separate bowl, whisk together the juice of the remaining lemon, olive oil, white vinegar, salt, and pepper. Pour this dressing over the cucumber mixture and toss to combine.

6. Serve the lemon dill salmon hot with the refreshing cucumber salad on the side.

Nutrition Facts (per serving):

- Calories: 300
- Total Fat: 18g
- Saturated Fat: 3g
- Cholesterol: 80mg
- Sodium: 150mg
- Total Carbohydrate: 6g
- Dietary Fiber: 2g
- Sugars: 2g
- Protein: 28g

Note: The nutrition facts are approximate and may vary depending on the ingredients used.

BUFFALO CAULIFLOWER BITES

Prep Time: 15 minutes Cooking Time: 25 minutes Serving: 4 servings

Ingredients:

- One medium head of cauliflower, cut into florets
- 1 cup all-purpose flour
- 1 cup milk (or a non-dairy alternative)
- One teaspoon of garlic powder
- One teaspoon of onion powder
- 1/2 teaspoon smoked paprika
- 1/2 teaspoon salt
- 1/4 teaspoon black pepper
- 1 cup buffalo hot sauce
- Two tablespoons melted butter (or a non-dairy alternative)
- Ranch or blue cheese dressing for serving
- Celery sticks for serving

Directions:

1. Preheat your oven to 450°F (230°C). Line a baking sheet with parchment paper and set it aside.

2. In a large mixing bowl, whisk together the flour, milk, garlic powder, onion powder, smoked paprika, salt, and black pepper until you have a smooth batter.

3. Dip each cauliflower floret into the batter, ensuring it's evenly coated. Allow any excess batter to drip off, then place the coated floret onto the prepared baking sheet. Repeat with the remaining florets.

4. Bake the cauliflower in the preheated oven for 20-25 minutes or until golden brown and crispy.

5. While the cauliflower is baking, prepare the buffalo sauce. Mix the buffalo hot sauce and melted butter in a small bowl until well combined.

6. Once the cauliflower is cooked, remove it from the oven and let it cool for a few minutes. Transfer the baked cauliflower to a large mixing bowl.

7. Pour the buffalo sauce over the cauliflower and toss gently until all the florets are evenly coated.

8. Serve the buffalo cauliflower bites with ranch or blue cheese dressing on the side and celery sticks for dipping.

Nutrition Facts (per serving):

- Calories: 200
- Total Fat: 5g
- Saturated Fat: 2g
- Cholesterol: 10mg
- Sodium: 1000mg
- Total Carbohydrate: 35g
- Dietary Fiber: 4g
- Sugars: 3g
- Protein: 7g

Enjoy your delicious Buffalo Cauliflower Bites!

SPINACH AND RICOTTA STUFFED CHICKEN BREAST

Prep Time: 20 minutes Cooking Time: 35 minutes Serving: 4 servings

Ingredients:

- Four boneless, skinless chicken breasts

- 2 cups fresh spinach leaves
- 1 cup ricotta cheese
- 1/4 cup grated Parmesan cheese
- Two cloves garlic, minced
- One teaspoon of dried Italian seasoning
- Salt and pepper, to taste
- Two tablespoons of olive oil

Directions:

1. Preheat the oven to 375°F (190°C).

2. Using a sharp knife, make a horizontal cut in each chicken breast to create a pocket for the stuffing. Be careful not to cut all the way through.

3. In a mixing bowl, combine the spinach, ricotta cheese, Parmesan cheese, minced garlic, dried Italian seasoning, salt, and pepper. Mix well to combine.

4. Spoon the spinach and ricotta mixture into each chicken breast pocket, dividing it evenly among them.

5. Close the chicken breasts and secure them with toothpicks to prevent the stuffing from falling out.

6. Season the outside of the chicken breasts with salt and pepper.

7. Heat olive oil in an oven-safe skillet over medium-high heat. Once the oil is hot, add the stuffed chicken breasts to the skillet.

8. Sear the chicken breasts for about 3-4 minutes on each side until golden brown.

9. Transfer the skillet to the preheated oven and bake for 20-25 minutes or until the chicken is cooked through and no longer pink in the centre.

10. Remove the chicken from the oven and let it rest for a few minutes before serving.

11. Serve the spinach and ricotta stuffed chicken breasts as a main dish with a side of your choice, such as roasted vegetables or mashed potatoes.

Nutrition Facts: The nutrition information will vary depending on the specific brands and quantities of ingredients used. However, here is a general approximation for one serving of spinach and ricotta stuffed chicken breast:

Calories: 280 Total Fat: 14g

- Saturated Fat: 6g

- Trans Fat: 0g Cholesterol: 110mg Sodium: 360mg Total Carbohydrate: 5g
- Dietary Fiber: 1g
- Sugars: 2g Protein: 34g

Please note that these values are approximate and may vary based on the specific ingredients and cooking methods used.

BACON-WRAPPED CHICKEN SKEWERS

Prep Time: 20 minutes Cooking Time: 15 minutes Serving: 4 servings

Ingredients:

- Four boneless, skinless chicken breasts
- Eight slices of bacon
- 1/4 cup soy sauce
- Two tablespoons honey
- Two tablespoons of Dijon mustard
- Two cloves of garlic, minced
- One teaspoon of smoked paprika
- 1/2 teaspoon black pepper

- Wooden skewers, soaked in water for 30 minutes

Directions:

1. Preheat your grill to medium-high heat.

2. Cut the chicken breasts into 1-inch cubes.

3. In a bowl, whisk together the soy sauce, honey, Dijon mustard, minced garlic, smoked paprika, and black pepper.

4. Place the chicken cubes in the bowl with the marinade, and toss to coat evenly. Allow the chicken to marinate for at least 10 minutes.

5. While the chicken is marinating, cut each slice of bacon in half.

6. Wrap each chicken cube with half a slice of bacon, and thread them onto the soaked wooden skewers.

7. Once the grill is hot, place the bacon-wrapped chicken skewers on the grill grates. Cook for about 6-8 minutes per side, or until the bacon is crispy and the chicken is cooked through, reaching an internal temperature of 165°F (74°C).

8. Remove the skewers from the grill and let them rest for a few minutes before serving.

9. Serve the bacon-wrapped chicken skewers as an appetizer or main dish, and enjoy!

Nutrition Facts (per serving):

- Calories: 320
- Fat: 15g
- Protein: 30g
- Carbohydrates: 14g
- Fibre: 0.5g
- Sugar: 11g
- Sodium: 830mg

Note: The nutrition facts are approximate and may vary based on the specific ingredients used and serving size.

KETO-FRIENDLY CHILI

Prep Time: 15 minutes Cooking Time: 1-hour Servings: 6

Ingredients:

- 2 pounds of ground beef
- One medium onion, diced
- Three cloves garlic, minced
- One bell pepper, diced

- One jalapeno pepper, seeded and minced (optional, for heat)
- One can (14 ounces) of diced tomatoes
- One can (6 ounces) of tomato paste
- 1 cup beef broth
- Two tablespoons of chili powder
- One tablespoon cumin
- One teaspoon paprika
- 1/2 teaspoon dried oregano
- 1/2 teaspoon salt
- 1/4 teaspoon black pepper
- Optional toppings: shredded cheddar cheese, sour cream, chopped green onions

Directions:

1. In a large pot or Dutch oven, cook the ground beef over medium heat until browned. Drain excess fat if needed.

2. Add the diced onion, minced garlic, bell pepper, and jalapeno pepper to the pot. Cook for about 5 minutes until the vegetables are slightly softened.

3. Stir in the diced tomatoes, tomato paste, beef broth, chilli powder, cumin, paprika,

dried oregano, salt, and black pepper. Mix well to combine all the ingredients.

4. Bring the chilli to a boil, then reduce the heat to low. Cover and simmer for 45 minutes to 1 hour, stirring occasionally.

5. After the chilli has simmered, taste and adjust the seasonings if desired.

6. Serve the keto-friendly chilli hot in bowls and top with shredded cheddar cheese, sour cream, and chopped green onions if desired.

Nutrition Facts (per serving): Calories: 380 Total Fat: 26g

- Saturated Fat: 10g
- Trans Fat: 1g Cholesterol: 95mg Sodium: 550mg Total Carbohydrate: 8g
- Dietary Fiber: 2g
- Sugars: 4g Protein: 29g

Note: The nutrition facts are approximate and may vary based on the specific ingredients used.

PARMESAN ROASTED GREEN BEANS

Prep Time: 10 minutes Cooking Time: 15 minutes Serving: 4

Ingredients:

- 1 pound fresh green beans, ends trimmed
- Two tablespoons of olive oil
- 1/2 cup grated Parmesan cheese
- One teaspoon of garlic powder
- 1/2 teaspoon salt
- 1/4 teaspoon black pepper

Directions:

1. Preheat the oven to 425°F (220°C).

2. In a large bowl, toss the green beans with olive oil until they are well coated.

3. In a separate bowl, combine the Parmesan cheese, garlic powder, salt, and black pepper.

4. Sprinkle the Parmesan mixture over the green beans and toss until they are evenly coated.

5. Spread the green beans in a single layer on a baking sheet.

6. Roast in the preheated oven for 12-15 minutes or until the green beans are tender and the Parmesan is golden brown.

7. Remove from the oven and let them cool for a few minutes before serving.

Nutrition Facts: Here are the approximate nutrition facts per serving:

- Calories: 150
- Fat: 10g
- Saturated Fat: 3g
- Cholesterol: 10mg
- Sodium: 390mg
- Carbohydrates: 10g
- Fibre: 4g
- Sugar: 4g
- Protein: 7g

Note: Nutrition facts may vary depending on the specific ingredients used and any modifications made to the recipe.

COCONUT LIME CHICKEN CURRY

Prep Time: 15 minutes Cooking Time: 30 minutes Serving: 4 servings

Ingredients:

- 1.5 lbs (680g) boneless, skinless chicken breasts cut into bite-sized pieces
- One tablespoon of vegetable oil
- One large onion, diced
- Three cloves garlic, minced
- One tablespoon of grated ginger
- Two tablespoons of red curry paste
- One can (13.5 oz) of coconut milk
- Juice of 2 limes
- One tablespoon of fish sauce
- One tablespoon of brown sugar
- One red bell pepper, seeded and sliced
- 1 cup snap peas
- Fresh cilantro, chopped (for garnish)
- Cooked rice or naan bread (for serving)

Directions:

1. heat the vegetable oil over medium heat in a large skillet or wok. Add the diced onion and sauté until softened, about 5 minutes.

2. Add the minced garlic and grated ginger to the skillet and cook for another minute until fragrant.

3. Stir in the red curry paste and cook for another minute to release its flavours.

4. Add the chicken pieces to the skillet and cook until they are browned on all sides, about 5 minutes.

5. Pour in the coconut milk, lime juice, fish sauce, and brown sugar. Stir well to combine all the ingredients.

6. Bring the mixture to a simmer and let it cook for 10 minutes, allowing the flavours to meld together.

7. Add the sliced red bell pepper and snap peas to the skillet and cook for 5 minutes or until the vegetables are tender-crisp.

8. Taste the curry and adjust the seasoning according to your preference. You can add more lime juice, fish sauce, or sugar if desired.

9. Remove the skillet from the heat and garnish the curry with fresh cilantro.

10. Serve the Coconut Lime Chicken Curry over cooked rice or with naan bread.

Nutrition Facts (per serving):

- Calories: 320
- Total Fat: 15g
- Saturated Fat: 10g
- Cholesterol: 80mg
- Sodium: 550mg
- Carbohydrates: 15g
- Fibre: 3g
- Sugar: 6g
- Protein: 30g

Note: The nutrition facts are approximate and may vary depending on the ingredients used.

STUFFED BELL PEPPERS WITH GROUND BEEF AND CHEESE

Prep Time: 20 minutes Cooking Time: 40 minutes Serving: 4

Ingredients:

- Four large bell peppers (any colour)

- 1 pound (450 grams) of ground beef
- One small onion, diced
- Two cloves garlic, minced
- 1 cup cooked rice
- 1 cup tomato sauce
- 1/2 cup shredded cheddar cheese
- 1/2 cup shredded mozzarella cheese
- One teaspoon of dried oregano
- One teaspoon of dried basil
- Salt and pepper to taste
- Fresh parsley for garnish

Directions:

1. Preheat your oven to 375°F (190°C).

2. Cut off the tops of the bell peppers and remove the seeds and membranes from the inside. Rinse them under cold water and set them aside.

3. In a large skillet, cook the ground beef over medium heat until browned. Drain any excess fat.

4. Add the diced onion and minced garlic to the skillet with the ground beef. Cook for 2-3 minutes until the onion becomes translucent.

5. Stir in the cooked rice, tomato sauce, dried oregano, dried basil, salt, and pepper. Mix well and cook for another 2-3 minutes to allow the flavours to combine.

6. Fill each bell pepper with the ground beef mixture, pressing it down gently to fill the cavity.

7. Place the stuffed bell peppers in a baking dish and cover with aluminium foil. Bake in the preheated oven for 25 minutes.

8. After 25 minutes, remove the foil from the baking dish and sprinkle the shredded cheddar and mozzarella cheese evenly over the tops of the bell peppers.

9. Return the baking dish to the oven and bake for an additional 10-15 minutes or until the cheese is melted and lightly golden.

10. Once cooked, remove the stuffed bell peppers from the oven and let them cool for a few minutes. Garnish with fresh parsley.

11. Serve the stuffed bell peppers hot, and enjoy!

Nutrition Facts (per serving):

- Calories: 375
- Total Fat: 18g

- Saturated Fat: 8g
- Cholesterol: 79mg
- Sodium: 598mg
- Carbohydrates: 24g
- Fibre: 4g
- Sugar: 8g
- Protein: 27g

Note: Nutritional values may vary depending on the specific ingredients and brands used.

GARLIC BUTTER STEAK BITES

Prep Time: 15 minutes Cooking Time: 10 minutes Serving: 4 servings

Ingredients:
- 1 lb (450 g) sirloin steak, cut into bite-sized cubes
- Four tablespoons of unsalted butter
- Four cloves garlic, minced
- One teaspoon of dried thyme
- Salt and black pepper, to taste

- Chopped fresh parsley for garnish (optional)

Directions:

1. In a large skillet, melt two tablespoons of butter over medium-high heat.

2. Add the minced garlic to the skillet and sauté for about 1 minute until fragrant.

3. Season the steak bites with salt, black pepper, and dried thyme. Add them to the skillet and cook for 2-3 minutes, stirring occasionally, until they are browned on all sides. Remove the steak bites from the skillet and set them aside.

4. In the same skillet, melt the remaining two tablespoons of butter over medium heat.

5. Add the cooked steak bites back to the skillet and toss them in the garlic butter sauce for an additional 1-2 minutes until they are cooked to your desired level of doneness.

6. Remove the skillet from heat and let the steak bites rest for a few minutes.

7. Garnish with chopped fresh parsley, if desired, before serving.

Nutrition Facts (per serving):

- Calories: 330
- Fat: 24g
- Saturated Fat: 12g
- Cholesterol: 105mg
- Sodium: 85mg
- Carbohydrates: 1g
- Protein: 26g

Note: The nutrition facts are approximate values and may vary depending on the specific ingredients used.

KETO EGGPLANT PARMESAN

Prep Time: 20 minutes Cooking Time: 45 minutes Serving: 4 servings

Ingredients:

- One large eggplant
- Salt
- 1 cup almond flour
- Two teaspoons of Italian seasoning
- One teaspoon of garlic powder
- Two large eggs
- 1 cup marinara sauce (sugar-free)

- 2 cups shredded mozzarella cheese
- Fresh basil leaves for garnish

Directions:

1. Preheat your oven to 375°F (190°C).

2. Slice the eggplant into 1/4-inch thick rounds. Sprinkle salt on both sides of each slice and place them in a colander for 15 minutes to release excess moisture. Rinse the slices and pat them dry with paper towels.

3. In a shallow bowl, combine the almond flour, Italian seasoning, and garlic powder. In another bowl, beat the eggs.

4. Dip each eggplant slice into the beaten eggs, allowing the excess to drip off, then coat it in the almond flour mixture. Shake off any excess coating and place the slices on a baking sheet lined with parchment paper.

5. Bake the coated eggplant slices for 20 minutes or until golden and crispy.

6. In a baking dish, spread a thin layer of marinara sauce on the bottom. Arrange half of the baked eggplant slices on top of the sauce. Spoon more marinara sauce over the eggplant slices and sprinkle with half of the shredded mozzarella cheese.

7. Repeat the previous step with the remaining eggplant slices, marinara sauce, and shredded mozzarella cheese.

8. Bake the assembled eggplant Parmesan in the oven for about 20-25 minutes or until the cheese is melted and bubbly.

9. Once cooked, remove from the oven and let it cool slightly. Garnish with fresh basil leaves.

10. Serve the Keto Eggplant Parmesan hot and enjoy!

Nutrition Facts (per serving):

- Calories: 280
- Fat: 19g
- Carbohydrates: 11g
- Fibre: 6g
- Protein: 18g
- Net Carbs: 5g

Note: The nutrition facts provided are estimates and may vary based on the specific ingredients used.

BAKED PARMESAN CRUSTED CHICKEN

Prep Time: 15 minutes Cooking Time: 25 minutes Serving: 4 servings

Ingredients:

- Four boneless, skinless chicken breasts
- 1 cup grated Parmesan cheese
- 1 cup breadcrumbs
- One teaspoon of garlic powder
- One teaspoon of dried oregano
- One teaspoon of dried basil
- 1/2 teaspoon salt
- 1/4 teaspoon black pepper
- Two eggs, beaten
- Cooking spray

Directions:

1. Preheat the oven to 400°F (200°C) and lightly grease a baking sheet with cooking spray.

2. In a shallow dish, combine the grated Parmesan cheese, breadcrumbs, garlic powder, dried oregano, dried basil, salt, and black pepper.

3. Dip each chicken breast into the beaten eggs, allowing any excess to drip off, then coat it thoroughly in the Parmesan mixture.

Press the mixture onto both sides of the chicken to ensure it adheres well.

4. Place the coated chicken breasts onto the prepared baking sheet. Repeat the process with the remaining chicken breasts.

5. Lightly spray the tops of the chicken breasts with cooking spray to help them brown and become crispy.

6. Bake in the preheated oven for 20-25 minutes or until the chicken is cooked through and the coating is golden brown.

7. Remove from the oven and let the chicken rest for a few minutes before serving.

8. Serve the Baked Parmesan Crusted Chicken with your favourite side dishes such as roasted vegetables, mashed potatoes, or a fresh salad.

Nutrition Facts (per serving):

- Calories: 320
- Total Fat: 11g
- Saturated Fat: 4g
- Cholesterol: 180mg
- Sodium: 760mg
- Total Carbohydrate: 15g

- Dietary Fiber: 1g
- Sugars: 1g
- Protein: 39g

Note: The nutrition facts are approximate and may vary depending on the specific ingredients and serving size.

BROCCOLI CHEDDAR STUFFED CHICKEN BREAST

Prep Time: 20 minutes Cooking Time: 30 minutes Serving: 4 servings

Ingredients:

- Four boneless, skinless chicken breasts
- 1 cup steamed broccoli florets, chopped
- 1 cup shredded cheddar cheese
- 1/2 teaspoon garlic powder
- 1/2 teaspoon onion powder
- 1/2 teaspoon paprika
- Salt and pepper to taste
- Two tablespoons of olive oil

Directions:

1. Preheat your oven to 375°F (190°C).

2. Slice each chicken breast horizontally to create a pocket without cutting through.

3. In a mixing bowl, combine the chopped broccoli, shredded cheddar cheese, garlic powder, onion powder, paprika, salt, and pepper. Mix well.

4. Spoon the broccoli and cheese mixture into the pocket of each chicken breast, dividing it equally among them.

5. Use toothpicks to secure the openings of the chicken breasts and hold the filling inside.

6. Heat the olive oil in an oven-safe skillet over medium-high heat.

7. Carefully place the stuffed chicken breasts into the skillet and cook for 3-4 minutes on each side until golden brown.

8. Transfer the skillet to the preheated oven and bake for about 20 minutes or until the chicken is cooked through and no longer pink in the centre.

9. Once cooked, remove the toothpicks from the chicken breasts.

10. Serve the broccoli cheddar stuffed chicken breasts hot with your favourite side dishes.

Nutrition Facts (per serving):

- Calories: 320
- Total Fat: 16g
- Saturated Fat: 7g
- Cholesterol: 105mg
- Sodium: 330mg
- Carbohydrates: 3g
- Fibre: 1g
- Sugars: 1g
- Protein: 40g

Enjoy your delicious broccoli cheddar stuffed chicken breasts!

BACON-WRAPPED SHRIMP

Prep Time: 15 minutes Cooking Time: 15 minutes Servings: 4

Ingredients:

- 16 large shrimp, peeled and deveined
- Eight slices of bacon

- Two tablespoons of olive oil
- Two tablespoons honey
- One tablespoon of lemon juice
- One teaspoon of smoked paprika
- Salt and black pepper to taste
- Wooden toothpicks

Directions:

1. Preheat your oven to 400°F (200°C).

2. In a small bowl, whisk together the olive oil, honey, lemon juice, smoked paprika, salt, and black pepper.

3. Take a shrimp and wrap it with a slice of bacon, securing the bacon with a wooden toothpick. Repeat with the remaining shrimp and bacon.

4. Place the bacon-wrapped shrimp in a baking dish and brush them with the prepared olive oil mixture, making sure to coat them evenly.

5. Bake the shrimp in the oven for about 12-15 minutes, or until the bacon is crispy and the shrimp are cooked through. You can also broil them for the last 2-3 minutes to get an extra crispy bacon.

6. Once cooked, remove the toothpicks from the shrimp.

7. Serve the bacon-wrapped shrimp hot as an appetizer or a main course with your favourite dipping sauce or a side of salad.

Nutrition Facts (per serving):

- Calories: 245
- Fat: 14g
- Saturated Fat: 4g
- Cholesterol: 145mg
- Sodium: 560mg
- Carbohydrates: 7g
- Fibre: 0g
- Sugar: 6g
- Protein: 21g

Note: The nutrition facts are approximate and may vary depending on the specific ingredients and quantities used.

CAULIFLOWER SHEPHERD'S PIE

Prep Time: 20 minutes Cooking Time: 40 minutes Serving: 6 servings

Ingredients:

- One large head of cauliflower, cut into florets
- Two tablespoons butter
- 1/4 cup milk (any type you prefer)
- Salt and pepper, to taste
- Two tablespoons of olive oil
- One onion, chopped
- Two carrots, peeled and diced
- Two cloves garlic, minced
- 1 pound ground beef (or ground turkey for a lighter version)
- One teaspoon dried thyme
- One teaspoon dried rosemary
- 1 cup frozen peas
- 1 cup beef or vegetable broth
- Two tablespoons tomato paste
- One tablespoon Worcestershire sauce
- 1 cup shredded cheddar cheese

Directions:

1. Preheat your oven to 400°F (200°C).

2. Place the cauliflower florets in a large pot of salted water and boil them. Cook for about

10 minutes or until the cauliflower is tender. Drain the cauliflower and transfer it to a large bowl.

3. Add the butter, milk, salt, and pepper to the bowl with the cauliflower. Use a potato masher or immersion blender to mash the cauliflower until it reaches a mashed potato-like consistency. Set aside.

4. Heat the olive oil in a large skillet over medium heat. Add the chopped onion and diced carrots, and cook for about 5 minutes or until they soften. Add the minced garlic and cook for an additional 1 minute.

5. Add the ground beef to the skillet and cook until browned, breaking it up with a spoon as it cooks. Stir in the dried thyme, rosemary, frozen peas, beef or vegetable broth, tomato paste, and Worcestershire sauce. Simmer for 10 minutes, allowing the flavours to meld together. Season with salt and pepper to taste.

6. Transfer the beef mixture to a baking dish and spread it evenly. Spoon the mashed cauliflower over the top and spread it out to cover the beef completely.

7. Sprinkle the shredded cheddar cheese on top of the cauliflower layer.

8. Place the baking dish in the preheated oven and bake for 20 minutes or until the cheese is melted and bubbling.

9. Remove from the oven and let it cool for a few minutes before serving.

Nutrition Facts: (The following nutritional information is approximate and may vary depending on the ingredients used)

- Calories: 320
- Total Fat: 19g
- Saturated Fat: 9g
- Cholesterol: 75mg
- Sodium: 450mg
- Total Carbohydrate: 16g
- Dietary Fiber: 4g
- Sugars: 6g
- Protein: 23g

Enjoy your delicious Cauliflower Shepherd's Pie!

LEMON GARLIC HERB ROASTED PORK TENDERLOIN

Prep Time: 15 minutes Cooking Time: 25 minutes Serving: 4 servings

Ingredients:

- 1.5 pounds of pork tenderloin
- Three cloves garlic, minced
- Two tablespoons fresh lemon juice
- Two teaspoons lemon zest
- One tablespoon fresh rosemary, chopped
- One tablespoon fresh thyme leaves
- One teaspoon salt
- 1/2 teaspoon black pepper
- Two tablespoons olive oil

Directions:

1. Preheat your oven to 425°F (220°C).

2. In a small bowl, combine the minced garlic, lemon juice, lemon zest, rosemary, thyme, salt, black pepper, and olive oil. Mix well to make a marinade.

3. Place the pork tenderloin in a baking dish and pour the marinade over it. Make sure the tenderloin is evenly coated with the marinade.

4. Let the pork tenderloin marinate for about 10 minutes to absorb the flavours.

5. Once marinated, transfer the pork tenderloin to a baking sheet lined with foil or parchment paper.

6. Roast the pork in the preheated oven for 20-25 minutes or until the internal temperature reaches 145°F (63°C).

7. Remove the pork from the oven and let it rest for 5 minutes before slicing.

8. Slice the pork tenderloin into medallions and serve with your favourite sides or vegetables.

Nutrition Facts (per serving):

- Calories: 250
- Fat: 12g
- Protein: 32g
- Carbohydrates: 2g
- Fibre: 0.5g

Note: The nutrition facts may vary depending on the specific ingredients and portion sizes used.

CHEESY SPINACH STUFFED CHICKEN BREAST

Prep Time: 15 minutes Cooking Time: 25 minutes Serving: 4

Ingredients:

- Four boneless, skinless chicken breasts
- 1 cup fresh spinach, chopped
- 1 cup shredded mozzarella cheese
- 1/4 cup grated Parmesan cheese
- 1/4 cup cream cheese
- Two cloves garlic, minced
- One teaspoon dried oregano
- 1/2 teaspoon salt
- 1/2 teaspoon black pepper
- Two tablespoons olive oil

Directions:

1. Preheat your oven to 375°F (190°C).

2. Using a sharp knife, carefully cut a slit lengthwise in each chicken breast to create a pocket for the stuffing. Be careful not to cut all the way through.

3. In a mixing bowl, combine the chopped spinach, mozzarella cheese, Parmesan cheese, cream cheese, minced garlic, dried oregano, salt, and black pepper. Mix well until all the ingredients are evenly incorporated.

4. Stuff each chicken breast with the spinach and cheese mixture, pressing it down gently to ensure it fills the pocket evenly.

5. Heat the olive oil in an oven-safe skillet over medium-high heat. Once hot, add the stuffed chicken breasts to the skillet and sear them for 2-3 minutes on each side until they turn golden brown.

6. Transfer the skillet to the preheated oven and bake for 18-20 minutes until the chicken is cooked through and reaches an internal temperature of 165°F (74°C).

7. Remove the skillet from the oven and let the chicken rest for a few minutes before serving.

8. Slice the stuffed chicken breasts diagonally and serve them warm. You can garnish with additional grated Parmesan cheese and fresh parsley if desired.

Nutrition Facts (per serving):

- Calories: 320
- Fat: 16g
- Saturated Fat: 7g
- Cholesterol: 120mg
- Sodium: 540mg
- Carbohydrates: 2g
- Fibre: 1g
- Sugar: 1g
- Protein: 41g

Note: The nutrition facts are approximate and may vary depending on the ingredients used.

KETO CHICKEN ALFREDO

Prep Time: 10 minutes Cooking Time: 20 minutes Servings: 4

Ingredients:

- Four boneless, skinless chicken breasts
- Salt and pepper, to taste
- Two tablespoons olive oil
- Four cloves garlic, minced
- 1 cup heavy cream
- 1/2 cup grated Parmesan cheese
- 1/4 cup unsalted butter
- 1/4 teaspoon nutmeg
- Fresh parsley, chopped (for garnish)

Directions:

1. Season the chicken breasts with salt and pepper on both sides.

2. heat the olive oil over medium-high heat in a large skillet. Add the chicken breasts and cook for about 6-8 minutes per side or until they are cooked through and golden brown. Remove the chicken from the skillet and set aside.

3. In the same skillet, add the minced garlic and sauté for about 1 minute, until fragrant.

4. Reduce the heat to low and add the heavy cream, Parmesan cheese, butter, and nutmeg to the skillet. Stir well until the sauce is

smooth and creamy. Cook for about 3-4 minutes, stirring occasionally.

5. Slice the cooked chicken breasts into thin strips and add them to the skillet with the Alfredo sauce. Stir to coat the chicken with the sauce and cook for another 2 minutes, until heated through.

6. Remove the skillet from the heat and let the sauce thicken slightly.

7. Serve the Keto Chicken Alfredo hot, garnished with chopped fresh parsley.

Nutrition Facts (per serving):

- Calories: 450
- Fat: 34g
- Protein: 32g
- Carbohydrates: 2g
- Fibre: 0g
- Net Carbs: 2g

Note: The nutrition facts are approximate and may vary depending on the specific ingredients and quantities used.

CONCLUSION

Congratulations on completing the "Keto Diet Cookbook For Beginners: A Comprehensive Guide to Jumpstart Your Ketogenic Journey and Achieve Optimal Health and Weight Loss." You have taken an important step towards transforming your lifestyle and improving your well-being through the power of the ketogenic diet.

Throughout this ebook, we have explored the science behind the ketogenic diet, providing a solid understanding of how it works and why it can be beneficial for weight loss and overall health. We have covered the essential macronutrients and micronutrients to consider, as well as different variations of the ketogenic diet to suit your preferences and goals.

Moreover, we have equipped you with various delicious and easy-to-follow recipes specifically tailored for beginners. From hearty breakfast options to satisfying lunch and dinner ideas and even indulgent snacks and desserts, you now have a diverse range of culinary delights to enjoy while staying on track with your keto lifestyle.

In addition to the recipes, we have addressed common challenges and provided practical tips to help you overcome obstacles along the way. Whether it's managing keto flu symptoms, staying motivated, or navigating social situations, you now have a toolbox of strategies to ensure your success on the ketogenic journey.

Remember, the ketogenic diet is not just a short-term solution but a sustainable and long-lasting lifestyle change. It's about nourishing your body with wholesome, nutrient-dense foods while enjoying the benefits of increased energy, improved mental clarity, and weight loss.

As you move forward, continue to listen to your body, make adjustments as needed, and stay connected to the keto community for support and inspiration. Remember that everyone's journey is unique, and finding what works best for you is essential.

We hope this ebook has provided you with the knowledge, guidance, and inspiration you need to embark on a successful ketogenic journey. Embrace the power of ketosis, explore the incredible flavours and benefits of the ketogenic diet, and unlock your full potential for optimal health and weight loss.

Wishing you all the best on your keto adventure!

Made in United States
North Haven, CT
28 November 2024

61111198R00095